Grow Your Own Pharmacy

Grow Your Own Pharmacy

Linda Gray

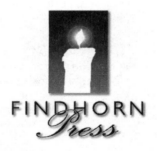

FINDHORN
Press

First published by Findhorn Press 2007

ISBN: 978-1-84409-089-1

British Library Cataloguing-in-Publication Data.
A catalogue record for this book is available from the British Library.

Edited by Shari Mueller and David Shaw
Cover design by Damian Keenan
Layout by Pam Bochel
Printed and bound by WS Bookwell, Finland

1 2 3 4 5 6 7 8 9 10 11 12 13 12 11 10 09 08 07

Published by
Findhorn Press
305A The Park,
Findhorn, Forres
Scotland IV36 3TE

Tel 01309 690582
Fax 01309 690036
email: info@findhornpress.com
www.findhornpress.com

Table of Contents

Introduction

Sugars – Natural and Processed

If you have ever strolled around a lovingly kept garden, whether it is full of fruits, vegetables, herbs or flowers, you may have experienced a sense of wonder, a sense of being at one with nature and an incredible feeling of being in touch with reality. Rushing around a supermarket grabbing packaged fruits and vegetables and all manner of processed foods just doesn't create that same warm, fuzzy feeling!

A high percentage of medical conditions are a direct result of our diet; we are what we eat after all. Personally I'd rather be seen as an exotic fruit salad than a burger, but then to each her own. It is, however, important to realise that what we eat has an effect on our body. Every action causes an equal and opposite reaction, that's just simple logic or cosmic law, however you look at it.

After reading hundreds if not thousands of articles and books about health, diet and weight problems, I arrived at the conclusion that a lot of serious medical conditions are a result of eating too much of the wrong foods. Obvious – yes. But listening to people talking about their diabetes or weight problems, or observing what they put in their supermarket carts, it appears we may understand the concept but we don't put the solutions into practice.

All those processed foods and yummy chocolate bars are just too appealing in their bright coloured packages with their 'reduced fat' claims. The fat may be reduced, but just check out the sugar and salt content…horrendous!

I recently read an enlightening book by Lee Janogly called *Only Fat People Skip Breakfast*. Over and over it emphasised the high sugar content in processed foods and suggested avoiding sugar in processed foods for one month. This sounds easy unless you are totally addicted to sugary snacks, as many people are, but I decided to try it.

I watched everything that I consumed over 30 days and ate only fresh foods, nothing processed. I limited my carbohydrate intake after breakfast and lost 14 pounds in one month without any effort – 14 pounds I needed to lose! The first few days I was a little irritable because I missed the taste of sugar and all the other goodies that are so bad for you.

The wonderful thing about fresh fruit and vegetables is that they contain natural sugar, and in fact, it's all the sugar we need to survive – the rest is surplus and causes many health concerns including heart disease, diabetes and obesity in a huge percentage of the western population.

In regions where processed foods aren't the norm, there are far less of these medical conditions – there may be other problems, but not these.

With all the scientific knowledge and information freely available to each and every one of us, we can and should make educated choices for our own well being. Growing our own vegetables and fruit is a huge step towards a healthy body, mind and spirit.

The Race for Cash

Before the middle of the twentieth century there were far fewer processed foods available and farming methods were simpler. Since then, the race to beat inflation, the rush to make as much money as possible, and the need to produce instant meals for our families have left us in a state of deficiency.

This has proved to be lucrative for the supplement and diet product industry. The consequence is that the average person is under stress to work longer hours to pay for the products he needs to make up for the deficiencies in his daily diet. More stress equals more need for supplements and various drugs to sort out the problems. This vicious circle many of us are racing around isn't actually helping the human race progress any further; it is in fact, stunting our growth and development. More illness means more precious resources needed to deal with the problems. Lack of development and growth causes more stress in the long term.

Not only are we not getting what we need from simple, everyday food which requires the use of supplements to balance our diet, but every time we buy a packaged product we are also helping to destroy the planet. Okay we can't be expected to put down tools and start living in caves, but we can make the effort to correct some of the wrongs and environmental crimes that have been committed over the past fifty years.

Back to the Future

We are here to nourish nature as nature nourishes us. A small plot of land for every family on the planet is all we really need to keep ourselves healthy and strong in mind, body and soul.

Intense farming methods of the past few decades have encouraged us to lose our sense of responsibility to the land and eventually the land will lose it's responsibility towards us if we don't get our act together soon. The organic associations and movements around the world are now finally being heard and their environmental knowledge is being taken up by some of the more progressive heads of state and governments.

Let's take a step back in time armed with all the knowledge and information available to us today, and get it right this time. To truly grow organic we have to start with the growing medium itself and correct the damage we've done to the soil.

Obviously no individual, however well meaning, can resolve this problem for the entire planet. But by attending to our own back yards, not only can we feed ourselves and our families better than ever before, but we may also be able to cut down on our working hours because less money will need to be earned.

This could very realistically have a positive effect and create more jobs, as well as setting an example to friends, friends of friends and eventually the whole world.

To get the condition of our growing medium well balanced, we can use technology. Get your soil tested and find out what chemicals have been used on it and what you can do to correct the problems.

Nourish for Life

Our bodies are living organisms just like plants. If we don't nourish a plant with the water and minerals from the soil, the plant will die. The same goes for all living creatures on the planet. We need the right input to gain the right output.

When you grow your own garden, the vegetables you harvest have been fully nourished, watered and cared for until the time when they are ready to nourish another living entity – you! The plants have taken minerals and vitamins from the soil and wondrously transformed them into healthful food. But if the soil isn't up to scratch and doesn't contain the minerals it needs to grow our fruit and vegetables, we won't be getting the full benefits that we need.

If we are ever going to get out of the pharmacy we have to get into the garden and take control…be the master or mistress of our own piece of land, however small. We don't have to have a gazebo, a water feature or the latest new variety of rose bush. That would be nice, but there are plenty of other good things to do with the space we have. Not only will that precious piece of land provide a healthy diet for you and your family, it will also give you some wonderful exercise. The point is, it should be enjoyed – whether you see it as a chore or a hobby – and it is ultimately going to keep you happy, healthy, and living longer.

Keep it Simple

Plan your garden to grow the vegetables you need. I've heard a number of people say "There's no point in growing tomatoes because when they are ready to pick in my garden the market is selling them at ridiculously low prices." Forget about the price. That's irrelevant for our discussion here. The main purpose of this book is to help you grow what you need from your land and to eat your homegrown, organic vegetables on a daily basis. Vegetables that have been stored under fluorescent lights in a supermarket will not have the same vitamin and mineral content as the same vegetables picked from your garden and eaten the same day.

Make notes as you read through this book, and tie in the foods your family likes to eat. There's absolutely no point in wasting time and energy growing lines of beetroot, however nutritious it is, if no one in the house will eat it. Of course, you could exchange with your neighbour or sell excess produce at a farmer's market, but that's the subject for another book! What we want to do is feed our families and feed them well.

Chapter One

Ingredients for a Healthy Body

These are nine of the most common vitamins that should be present in our daily diet. All of these vitamins can be produced from everyday fruit and vegetables and can be grown in an average garden with a little careful planning.

RDA Table (or RDI – recommended daily intake)		
	Female RDA	Male RDA
Vitamin A	700mcg.	900mcg.
Thiamine (B1)	1.1mg.	1.2mg.
Riboflavin (B2)	1.1mg.	1.3mg.
Vitamin B6	1.3mg.	1.3mg.
Vitamin C	40mg.–60mg.	40mg.–60mg.
Vitamin E	Approx. 3mg.	Approx. 4mg.
Niacin (B3)	13mg.	17mg.
Folate	Approx. 200mcg.	Approx. 200mcg.
Pantothenic Acid (B5)	Approx. 5.0mg.	Approx. 5.0mg.

Vitamin B12 and vitamin D are two very important vitamins to maintain a healthy body. These two vitamins are present in animal and dairy products as well as in light and sunshine and will not be part of this book.

RDA Table (or RDI – recommended daily intake for B12 and D vitamins)		
	Female RDA	Male RDA
Vitamin B12	1.0mcg. –1.5mcg.	1.0mcg. –1.5mcg.
Vitamin D	Approx. 5.0mcg.	Approx. 5.0mcg.

Vitamin A

Vitamin A acts as an antioxidant, neutralising free radicals when necessary. It is fat soluble and is stored in the body, mostly in the liver. Too much vitamin A is not good for the body and can result in fatigue and blurred vision. Too little vitamin A can result in unhealthy skin, wounds healing slowly and serious eye conditions. Vitamin A is needed for good vision, healthy skin and normal bone development. Carrots are the most common source of vitamin A. One medium-sized carrot will provide nearly all your daily recommended allowance. Generally, 50–200g. of source food provides approximately 150mcg. of vitamin A.

Good sources include:

- Apricots
- Artichokes
- Broccoli
- Brussels sprouts
- Cabbage
- Cantaloupe
- Carrots
- Cherries
- Cos lettuce (romaine)
- French beans
- Garlic
- Kale
- Onions
- Peppers
- Pumpkins
- Runner beans
- Spinach
- Sweet potatoes
- Tomatoes
- Turnip greens
- Watercress

Vitamin B1

Vitamin B1 converts carbohydrates and fats into energy. It helps the heart, digestive and nervous systems to function properly. Vitamin B1 cannot be stored in the body and should be replenished on a daily basis. A deficiency of vitamin B1 is rare but can occur in people who have a high alcohol intake; they will show symptoms such as poor appetite, fatigue and weight loss. 25–100g. of the source food will provide approx. 0.1 mg. of vitamin B1.

Good sources include:

- Artichokes
- Cabbage
- Carrots
- Cauliflower
- Celeriac
- Chicory
- Endive
- Garlic
- Leeks
- Mushrooms
- Nuts
- Onions
- Parsnips
- Peas
- Potatoes
- Pumpkins
- Seeds
- Soya beans (soy beans)
- Spinach
- Swedes (rutabagas)
- Sweet corn
- Watercress
- Whole grains and wholemeal products

Vitamin B2

Vitamin B2 is a little known vitamin that does a lot. It is essential in normal growth development and releases the energy from carbohydrates. Lack of vitamin B2 can result in anaemia, sore throats, mouth ulcers, dry skin and even eye sensitivity to bright lights. Milk and yoghurt are the most common source of vitamin B2. Between 85 and 300g. of source food provides 0.1mg. of vitamin B2.

Good sources include:

- Artichokes
- Asparagus
- Broccoli
- Garlic
- Mushrooms
- Okra
- Onions
- Salsify
- Spinach
- Turnip greens
- Whole grains

Vitamin B6

Vitamin B6 helps manufacture antibodies to fight infection and, as with all the B vitamins, B6 plays a major role in keeping blood cells acting efficiently. There are medical conditions that naturally decrease the amount of B6 in the blood, such as asthma, kidney disease and diabetes. Symptoms of a mild B6 deficiency include cracked lips, nausea and diarrhoea. A more severe deficiency could result in loss of appetite, anxiety and depression. A particularly good source of vitamin B6 is bananas. 100–250g of food source will provide 0.5mg. of vitamin B6.

Good sources include:

- Aubergine (eggplant)
- Bananas
- Beetroot
- Broccoli
- Cantaloupes
- Cauliflower
- Celeriac
- Courgette (zucchini)
- Grapes
- Green cabbage
- Leeks
- Legumes
- Mushrooms
- Nuts
- Parsnips
- Potatoes
- Raspberries
- Red peppers
- Shallots
- Spinach
- Sweet potatoes
- Squash
- Swedes (rutabagas)
- Sweet corn
- Tomatoes
- Turnips
- Watercress
- Whole grains

Vitamin C

Vitamin C is perhaps the most well known vitamin and the most unstable; it is often destroyed through cooking and food processing. Vitamin C is a healing vitamin and should be taken in larger doses when the body needs to repair itself after injury or illness; it improves resistance to infection. Lack of vitamin C results in many ailments including weakness, easily bruised skin, slow healing of wounds and in more severe cases, fatigue and depression. 50–200g. of food source provides at least 10mg. of vitamin C.

Good sources include:

- Apples
- Artichokes
- Asparagus
- Blackberries
- Broccoli
- Brussels sprouts
- Cabbage
- Carrots
- Cauliflower
- Celeriac
- Chicory
- Citrus fruits
- Courgettes (zucchini)
- Endive
- Fennel bulbs
- French beans
- Kale
- Kiwi fruit
- Leeks
- Lettuce
- Melons
- Onions
- Parsley
- Parsnips
- Pears
- Peas
- Peppers
- Radish
- Rhubarb
- Runner beans
- Shallots
- Spinach
- Squash
- Strawberries
- Swedes (rutabagas)
- Sweet corn
- Tomatoes
- Turnips
- Watercress

Vitamin E

Vitamin E is considered to be one of nature's best antioxidants protecting the body against free radicals. Long-term illness can cause deficiency of vitamin E. Deficiency symptoms include anaemia and problems with the nervous system; however, it is rare in a healthy body. 25–50g. of food source will provide 0.5mg. of vitamin E.

Good sources include:

- Blueberries
- Green leafy vegetables
- Kale
- Soya beans (soy beans)
- Sunflower seeds
- Wheat germ

Niacin (B3)

Niacin isn't talked about much but is one of the most active vitamins in the body. It breaks down fats and sugars and helps to maintain efficient functioning of the stomach, nervous system and skin. Niacin is found in protein-rich foods such as meat, fish and pulses (legumes). If these form a large part of our diet, niacin deficiency is unlikely to occur. Symptoms of niacin deficiency may include weakness and loss of appetite. More severe symptoms can include diarrhoea, skin rashes and inflammation in the mouth and tongue. Between 25 and 100g. of source food provides 1.0 mg. of niacin.

Good sources include:

- Artichokes
- Leafy green vegetables
- Mushrooms
- Parsley
- Peas
- Soya beans (soy beans)
- Sweet corn

Folate

Yet another of the B vitamins, folate (also called folic acid), isn't made by the body and must come from a good food source. Anaemia, fatigue, unhealthy weight loss and heartburn can be a result of folate deficiency. Eating less processed foods and remembering to eat 5 or more servings of fresh fruits and vegetables daily should prevent any folate deficiency. 85–200g. of food source will provide 30mcg. of folate.

Good sources include:

- Asparagus
- Blackberries
- Black-eyed beans (black-eyed peas)
- Broccoli
- Brussels sprouts
- Cabbage
- Cauliflower
- Celeriac
- Cos Lettuce (romaine)
- Courgette (zucchini)
- Fennel bulbs
- French beans
- Kidney beans
- Leafy green vegetables
- Leeks
- Legumes
- Lentils
- Mushrooms

- Oranges
- Parsnips
- Peas
- Raspberries
- Runner beans
- Salsify
- Spinach
- Squash
- Sweet corn

Pantothenic Acid (B5)

Pantothenic acid is a B-complex vitamin that helps to break down fats, proteins and carbohydrates and enables energy production. It is needed to produce B12 and helps maintain cell structure in the blood. It is unusual to be deficient in this vitamin but when it does occur it's usually as a result of a deficiency in all the B complex vitamins. Symptoms are normally fatigue and pain in the stomach. Pantothenic acid can be found in avocados and 100–250g. of food source will provide 0.5mg. of pantothenic acid.

Good sources include:

- Artichokes
- Avocado
- Broad beans
- Broccoli
- Chicory
- Haricot beans
- Lentils
- Mushrooms
- Sweet potatoes

Chapter Two

Introduction to Gardening

Gardening is fast becoming the world's number one hobby – and with good reason. Gardening will help you:

- keep fit and healthy with regular exercise in the fresh air
- enjoy quality time with the family – everyone can do it
- provide the best possible food for your daily needs

Gardening doesn't have to be hard work. Even if you are physically disabled or challenged, there are options. Does your budget allow you to employ someone to do the heavy work? Or perhaps you could offer a helpful soul some of the harvest in return for a little digging now and then? How about container gardening? Most plants can be successfully grown in pots and planters. Or try using the raised bed system.

Whichever method of gardening is best for you, you can start today. Collect some seed catalogues, browse through the glorious pictures and determine to produce the same!

The next few pages will help you decide what you need to start growing fresh produce for you and your family.

Gardening Tools

Whatever type of gardening you are planning on, a certain number of tools will be needed. If you have a large budget and are intending to go for it on a grand scale, then buy what you like. But if you are a little cautious or planning a smaller garden, you don't need to spend a lot.

If your land hasn't been worked before or has recently been cleared of trees and brambles, it's best to get the ground ploughed first. Make friends with a local farmer and offer him a bottle of wine to bring his tractor round and manoeuvre it over your land. This is how it's done in France anyway! If there aren't any tractors or farmers in your area, consider doing it yourself. Examine the land, decide what machine is necessary and get down to your local machinery rental shop.

A rotavator may be all you need to get the land ready to work on. If this work is too heavy for you, call in the experts, or change your plan…consider container plants or raised beds.

Basic Gardening Tools

The basic tools needed once you've got your workable space in the garden are:

- spade
- fork
- rake
- trowel
- watering can with a rosette attachment

It's surprising what you can achieve with only these few basic tools – you don't need to spend a lot of money for a simple garden.

Check on weight and size before you buy tools. Some tools are heavy and will contribute to backache and fatigue a lot sooner than a smaller, lighter tool would. Look at lengths of handles. If you're 6 ft. tall, you will be bending over more than someone who is 5 ft. tall using the same tool. Get the feel of the tool in the shop before you buy if at all possible. Choose tools that feel comfortable in your hand and have a solid feel to them. A flimsy tool may bend on contact with hard ground and can cause accidents.

Extra Safety Notes

- Garden overalls are practical and will protect your clothes.
- Gardening gloves are a must-have. They protect your hands from nettles, brambles, staining from certain plants and possible allergies.
- And steel-toe capped boots are 100% necessary to protect your feet if you plan to dig your garden or use large tools of any kind. Invest in a pair of decent, comfortable gardening boots and they will become your best friends.

Container Gardening

Larger tools won't be needed for simple container gardening. A larger-than-average trowel or a short handled spade or shovel could come in handy when filling pots with compost or soil, but otherwise, just a regular, sturdy trowel and your containers will get you started.

Other Garden Tools

Collect these tools as you need them and as they come to you. Car boot sales and flea markets are great places to find used tools that still have a lot of life in them at a reasonable price.

Shed ~ A garden shed is necessary to protect the tools and materials you need in the garden. As your hobby grows, so will the gardening bits and pieces, so investing in a shed space of some sort is really worthwhile before you even start gardening. I used an old caravan for a shed for many years. Paint it green or create an artistic landscape design so it blends into the garden nicely!

Greenhouse ~ A greenhouse will enable you to start seeds earlier than sowing directly outside. It doesn't have to be expensive either. Look out for discarded metal shed or greenhouse frames, and 'glaze' with a sheet of clear plastic. If you live in a moderate climate, a greenhouse is invaluable and will lengthen your growing season considerably.

Cloche ~ A cloche can be small – made from a couple of wire coat hangers and a sheet of clear plastic – or large – made from bendable plastic tubing or smooth willow branches bent into a tunnel shape – to protect your garden plants from the cold nights in spring and autumn. Cloches can be built from practically anything, depending on how creative you are. Make sure there aren't any sharp edges on the frame before you cover it in clear plastic. Secure the plastic with a couple of logs or large stones, so the wind doesn't take it away.

Poly-tunnels ~ If you have a large enough garden, a poly-tunnel is worth the investment. You can use them to lengthen your growing season. They are ideal to start off very early potatoes. In a poly-tunnel, potatoes can be started in late December and harvested in early spring. The only plants that don't particularly benefit from poly-tunnel or protected growing areas are kale, Brussels sprouts or parsnips, all of which are tastier after the first frost. The best sprouts I ever tasted were the ones I had to brush the snow from before picking.

Bits and Pieces

Recycle and benefit! Collect some of the following items during the year and keep them in the shed.

- Yoghurt and dessert containers (wash and dry well before storing) – these make handy pots for the gardener. Remember to punch a couple of holes in the bottom for drainage.
- Coat hangers and frames of almost any kind – could it be used for a cloche? Then keep it!
- Sheets of clear plastic – always useful if you live in a moderate climate and need to protect young plants from cold nights.
- Wooden or plastic trays – place a sheet of newspaper in the bottom and use for seed trays in the spring.
- Plastic paint trays – the kind you use with a roller. With a couple of holes punched in the bottom for drainage, these make perfect seed trays.
- Utensils – keep an old fork and spoon from the kitchen for dealing with any delicate operations in the greenhouse.
- Collect all plastic pots that can be recycled and used for potting your tomatoes later on – it's surprising how many you will need.

Compost Heap

Create a compost heap – you owe it to yourself and the planet to create one. Any natural foodstuffs must be recycled. It's almost criminal to put them in the bin. Vegetable peelings and leftovers (non-meat) are gold for the enthusiastic gardener.

Build a frame or buy a ready-made one, and start filling it. Keep it covered with anything suitable and all those leftovers and peelings will rot down all on their own and produce a beautiful, rich compost you can use for the next growing cycle in the garden. There are many places on the internet or books in the library that explain the process.

Don't keep the compost too near the house as any rotting material will smell at times and attract flies. Keep it covered to avoid these problems but inevitably there will be moments when it will smell a little. Tuck it away in an unused part of the garden, but remember to make it accessible. You need to be able to walk to the compost with a bowl of vegetable peelings, and you don't want to be climbing over bikes or cement mixers to get there.

About a year after you start your compost heap, the bottom layers will have already turned to soil. Dig this out, put through a garden sieve if necessary, and use for your young plants in the greenhouse, or dig it into the vegetable plot.

Preparing Your Growing Area

To be sure of producing the very best fruit and vegetables for your family, you will need to start at the beginning and get the soil checked. Have an analysis done by your local organic association or gardening centre if they provide the service or buy a soil testing kit and do it yourself. Take samples from different areas of your garden and avoid places where there has been a bonfire or compost heap or where you have mixed cement or fixed the car.

As long as no heavy chemicals have been spilled on your piece of land, you should be able to make up for any short fall. If your garden has been used for growing fruit and vegetables before, chances are it will be fine but an analysis will help you diagnose any problems that may occur. Cabbages, for example, don't do well in a highly acidic soil, but a little adjustment a few months before sowing can mean the difference between a poor crop and a rich one.

Test to see if you have acid, alkaline or neutral soil. An acid soil can be neutralised with calcified seaweed. General purpose organic fertilisers will restore the balance of nutrients in most soil. To make absolutely sure you have organic approved soil, you will need to get in touch with your local organic association who will be able to steer you in the right direction.

Dig in plenty of organic matter during the autumn to winter months and keep building your compost heap. Consider creating a comfrey feeder. Comfrey is a green manure that acts as a tonic to help release minerals into the soil so plants can absorb the nutrients they need easily and effectively. Comfrey will grow in shadier areas of your garden and is worth the space if you can afford it. Comfrey leaves can be harvested twice, sometimes three times a year and the plants can be grown under a hedgerow or next to a fence.

If you haven't the space to build a feeder, layer comfrey leaves into your compost heap as they become ready to harvest (just before flowering). Or use the leaves as mulch in the spring around your new plants. If you're planting potatoes, lay comfrey leaves in the trench and place the seed potatoes directly on the leaves. Potato plants benefit from the minerals and you will get a huge crop of potatoes.

If you do have the space for a comfrey feeder, use a barrel with a tap at the bottom and fill with comfrey leaves when they are available. Add some nettles if you don't have a lot of comfrey during the first few years. Place a filter behind the tap so the leaves don't clog it up when you come to pour off the liquid. After filling with leaves, weigh down with a heavy stone or other suitable weight and cover.

After a few weeks the leaves will have broken down. Place a watering can or mixing tub directly under the tap and release the fluid. Mix the comfrey fluid with water – about a 50–50 ratio and use to feed your fruit and vegetables. Pour onto the soil around the base of the plants so the soil absorbs it straight away. And if possible, apply on a dry day so the rain doesn't wash it away too soon. Warning: This liquid is very smelly and although it's a natural smell, it can be very strong. Not for the faint-hearted.

Use any spare patches of garden to produce organic material for your veggie beds. Compost heaps and green manures are so beneficial for a rich harvest of fresh, organic fruit and vegetables.

Planning the Garden Space

What do you want from your garden? Do you need to keep a play area for the children? Are you planning to have a water feature? Herb beds? Colourful flowering displays?

Make a few plans. Draw out some rough sketches on paper and give some thought to where your vegetable plot will be best situated. Watch where the sun comes up and which parts of your garden get the most sunlight throughout the day.

Do you have a sunroom or conservatory you can use for your plants? If not, choose the lightest room in the house and prepare a space specially for starting off seedlings, or use a greenhouse, poly-tunnel or cloche. Containers can be placed in sunny, warm spots around the garden or on the patio or balcony.

Plan your garden, and then define your vegetable plot. First put some lines up. Find sticks or tent pegs, and tie lengths of string to form a square or whatever shape you're planning on. Push the sticks firmly in the ground. Use a sharp spade and dig round the edge of your plot, following the string.

If the plot hasn't been worked before, dig out a trench about the depth of your spade and leave this soil at the side of your plot. Next dig over another spade depth within this trench and break the soil up with the edge of your spade or a fork. Then move back and dig over the next line and tip it straight into the lower level you just created. Dig the bottom of the trench. Remove any large rocks, debris or stubborn weeds as you go. This double digging method should be continued until you have prepared the whole vegetable plot. If you have organic matter to work into the ground, do it at the same time to avoid another digging session. Lay the matter onto the lower level after you have dug it and tip the soil from the next line over it. At the end, put the discarded soil from the first trench back into the final trench.

Preparing the soil in this way will ensure the ground is clean and fine enough for roots to develop and especially for root vegetables such as carrots. Once the double dig has been done initially it shouldn't be necessary to repeat for several years unless your soil is particularly heavy.

To Dig or not to Dig?

Digging can be therapeutic. I have worked out loads of stubborn problems while turning the earth, and there's nearly always a robin or two looking out for up-turned worms. Robins are great companions in the garden. However, if digging really isn't your thing, plan out some raised beds.

Raised beds are narrow strips of ground you never walk on. They should be measured so you can reach them from either side without stepping on the bed at all. After the first dig, they need very light forking every now and then, but never require a heavy digging session.

Plants can be grown much closer together in raised beds – the soil is finer, and the roots go deeper. Therefore you can grow more in a smaller space.

The Henry Doubleday Research Association, now known as Garden Organic, was a pioneer of raised beds and many organic gardeners around the world use this system.

Keeping Notes

It's always a good idea to keep a garden diary for future reference. Any kind of notebook will do. Draw out a sketch of your garden or make a list of your containers at the beginning of the book.

Keep regular notes on:
- what you did in the garden and on what date
- dates and names of seeds sown, and where (directly in the garden or in seed trays)
- dates you put out young plants
- any problems such as pests or viruses and how you treated them
- notable events such as a family of frogs moving in (frogs and toads are useful in your garden and you should welcome them, not necessarily with open arms, but definitely an open mind)
- weather conditions

What to Grow and Where

Read Chapters 4 to 14 on growing various herbs and vegetables to decide what your family likes to eat. Make some notes and jot down alternative produce just in case you get a crop failure – unfortunately it does happen. Nature can be tough sometimes and if you get a white butterfly attack on your cabbages and don't spot it in time, you can lose a whole crop over a couple of days.

Where to grow depends on the available space. You should generally look for the sunniest spots – out of any cross-winds – for regular outdoor planting.

Position greenhouses and poly-tunnels carefully. A little shade is useful – on long, sunny days, glass and plastic can become very hot and plants inside can burn or dry out very quickly. Glass structures can be whitewashed during very hot summers. Special covers can also be bought for covering plants in bright sunshine, and these work very well, but if you have a little natural shade that you can take advantage of, all the better. Reducing the cost and the amount of work involved is always pleasing.

Many plants, even potatoes, can be grown in containers. Gardeners will tell you planting potatoes involves a lot of heavy work but the end result is always worthwhile. That's very true, but you can grow potatoes in rubber tyres or other containers and you won't need to 'earth them up' every couple of weeks, or dig long trenches when you first plant them. And they taste just as good.

Herbs, tomatoes, peppers, aubergines and other similar crops are well adapted to container growing and the pots can be placed around the garden, conservatory, greenhouse or poly-tunnel according to their needs. Move into the sun for warmth, into the shade if too hot or into a sheltered spot if the weather takes a turn for the worse. The most important thing to remember with container growing is that the soil can dry out very quickly. Keep the soil moist at all times but never waterlogged. Make sure the containers you use are well-drained and water at least once a day during the growing season.

Seeds or Plants
Another choice to make. Try both. Start off some seeds early in the year and keep them warm and watered ready for planting out in the spring. Sowing from seed does keep you more in touch with the whole process and children love this part of the gardening journey. Make sure you start sowing seed early in the year, but only when you can keep the resulting seedlings warm enough.

If you don't have the time or space to be bothered with seeds, you will be able to buy most vegetable plants at a young stage in their development all ready to plant out in the garden at the right time. The only down side is that you won't get the choice of varieties you would from seed. It would be impossible for growers to provide all varieties, so they tend to stick with popular, easy-to-grow types. This is great for the new gardener, and you shouldn't have too many problems when you buy local, ready-started veggie plants, some places even have organic plants.

When you see tomato plants for sale, it's probably about the right time in your region for planting out tomatoes. Are yours ready? Root crops will need to be started from seed as they don't transplant well.

Chapter Three

Vitamin Content at a Glance

The everyday garden vegetables we are about to explore can all be grown in a moderate climate but some will need a little warmth and TLC to get them started.

Vitamin A ~ Carrots, Cos Lettuce, Kale, Pumpkin

Carrot ~ Properties
Carrots contain beta-carotene, which is a form of vitamin A. They also contain vitamins B1 and B6. Carrots can be eaten raw or cooked and make a great snack food. One medium carrot will provide enough vitamin A for an average adult per day. Children should be encouraged to eat raw carrot sticks in place of fast food snacks and even babies can be given carrot, although unless they have a full set of teeth, it's wiser to cook them first. Because of their sweet flavour, carrots also make great cakes.

Composition of carrots per 100g.

Nutrient		Unit	Raw	Cooked
Water		g.	88.29	90.17
Energy		calories	41	35
Protein		g.	0.93	0.76
Lipid (fat)		g.	0.24	0.18
Fibre		g.	2.8	3.0
Sugars (total)		g.	4.54	3.45
Minerals:	Calcium	mg.	33	30
	Iron	mg.	0.30	0.34
Vitamins:	Vitamin A	mcg.	841	860
	Vitamin B1	mg.	0.066	0.066
	Vitamin B2	mg.	0.058	0.044
	Vitamin B6	mg.	0.138	0.153
	Vitamin C	mg.	5.9	3.6
	Vitamin E	mg.	–	1.03
	Niacin	mg.	0.983	0.645
	Folate	mcg.	19	14
	Pantothenic Acid	mg.	0.273	0.232

Cos Lettuce (Romaine) ~ Properties

Cos or romaine lettuce has a high content of vitamins A and C and folate. The leaves have a thick rib down the centre, which is filled with a milky fluid. The ribs on the outer leaves are often slightly bitter and tend to be discarded when adding to the salad bowl. However, these leaves are the most nutritious part of the lettuce. The tips of cos lettuce are also sometimes bitter in taste but again they are high in vitamin content and should be eaten if possible. Adding a tasty salad dressing helps to balance the bitter taste.

Composition of cos lettuce per 100g.

Nutrient		Unit	Raw
Water		g.	94.61
Energy		calories	17
Protein		g.	1.23
Lipid (fat)		g.	0.30
Fibre		g.	2.1
Sugars (total)		g.	1.19
Minerals:	Calcium	mg.	33
	Iron	mg.	0.97
Vitamins:	Vitamin A	mcg.	290
	Vitamin B1	mg.	0.072
	Vitamin B2	mg.	0.067
	Vitamin B6	mg.	0.074
	Vitamin C	mg.	24.0
	Vitamin E	mg.	0.13
	Niacin	mg.	0.313
	Folate	mcg.	136
	Pantothenic Acid	mg.	0.142

Kale ~ Properties

Kale is a wonderful vegetable to grow for winter nourishment. It contains high doses of vitamin A, is a good source of vitamins C and E and is high in iron. Kale will grow in most moderate climates and will keep cropping from mid-winter right through to early spring. Because of its cold weather growing season, there are often less pests and diseases to worry about and kale will often just get on with growing all by itself, leaving you to enjoy it as you choose.

Composition of kale per 100g.

Nutrient	Unit	Raw	Cooked
Water	g.	84.46	91.20
Energy	calories	50	28
Protein	g.	3.30	1.90

Nutrient		Unit	Raw	Cooked
Lipid (fat)		g.	0.70	0.40
Fibre		g.	2.0	2.0
Sugars (total)		g.	No data	1.25
Minerals:	Calcium	mg.	135	72
	Iron	mg.	1.70	0.90
Vitamins:	Vitamin A	mcg.	769	681
	Vitamin B1	mg.	0.110	0.053
	Vitamin B2	mg.	0.130	0.070
	Vitamin B6	mg.	0.271	0.138
	Vitamin C	mg.	120.0	41.0
	Vitamin E	mg.	No data	0.85
	Niacin	mg.	1.000	0.500
	Folate	mcg.	29	13
	Pantothenic Acid	mg.	.0.091	0.049

Pumpkin ~ Properties

Pumpkins are 90% water but contain high quantities of vitamin A and other nutrients in their fleshy insides. Pumpkin seeds are high in minerals and are a good source of zinc. There are some who swear by pumpkin seeds as a prevention for osteoporosis and other major physical ailments. We are seeing more seeds of all sorts in our supermarkets these days, indicating we have finally accepted them as a healthy food.

Composition of pumpkin per 100g.

Nutrient		Unit	Roasted Seeds No Salt	Cooked Flesh
Water		g.	7.10	93.69
Energy		calories	522	20
Protein		g.	32.97	0.72
Lipid (fat)		g.	42.13	0.07
Fibre		g.	3.9	1.1
Sugars (total)		g.	1.00	1.02
Minerals:	Calcium	mg.	43	15
	Iron	mg.	14.94	0.57
Vitamins:	Vitamin A	mcg.	19	250
	Vitamin B1	mg.	0.210	0.031
	Vitamin B2	mg.	0.319	0.078
	Vitamin B6	mg.	0.090	0.044

Nutrient		Unit	Roasted Seeds No Salt	Cooked Flesh
	Vitamin C	mg.	1.8	4.7
	Vitamin E	mg.		0.80
	Niacin	mg.	1.742	0.413
	Folate	mcg.	57	9
	Pantothenic Acid	mg.	.0.339	0.201

Vitamin B1 ~ Broad beans, Garlic, Hazelnuts, Sweet corn

Broad Bean ~ Properties

The broad bean and many other beans are normally high in protein and vitamins and are a good, solid food to grow for the family. A grain is traditionally eaten with beans (beans on toast, dahl and rice etc.) because beans lack certain amino acids and grains help balance the meal.

Composition of broad beans per 100g.

Nutrient		Unit	Raw	Cooked
Water		g.	10.9	71.54
Energy		calories	341	110
Protein		g.	26.12	7.60
Lipid (fat)		g.	1.53	0.40
Fibre		g.	25.0	5.4
Sugars (total)		g.	5.70	1.82
Minerals:	Calcium	mg.	103	36
	Iron	mg.	6.70	1.50
Vitamins:	Vitamin A	mcg.	3	1
	Vitamin B1	mg.	0.555	0.097
	Vitamin B2	mg.	0.333	0.089
	Vitamin B6	mg.	0.366	0.072
	Vitamin C	mg.	1.4	0.3
	Vitamin E	mg.	0.05	0.02
	Niacin	mg.	2.832	0.711
	Folate	mcg.	423	104
	Pantothenic Acid	mg.	0.976	0.157

Garlic ~ Properties

Garlic has been known as a super healing herb for centuries. It's been used in herbal medicines to treat many ailments including the common cold. Garlic has been proved to be a powerful antibiotic, although it should never be taken in large doses. Garlic also has antioxidant effects, which help protect against free radicals. It is a good source of vitamin C and B vitamins. Chew parsley leaves to avoid 'garlic breath'.

Composition of garlic per 100g.

Nutrient		Unit	Raw
Water		g.	58.58
Energy		calories	149
Protein		g.	6.36
Lipid (fat)		g.	0.50
Fibre		g.	2.1
Sugars (total)		g.	1.00
Minerals:	Calcium	mg.	1.81
	Iron	mg.	1.70
Vitamins:	Vitamin A	mcg.	0
	Vitamin B1	mg.	0.200
	Vitamin B2	mg.	0.110
	Vitamin B6	mg.	1.235
	Vitamin C	mg.	31.2
	Vitamin E	mg.	0.01
	Niacin	mg.	1.700
	Folate	mcg.	3
	Pantothenic Acid	mg.	0.596

Hazelnut ~ Properties

All nuts are rich in protein, minerals and some vitamins. Some are higher in fat than others but all contain much needed fibre to keep the digestive system working well. Pecan nuts are known to help release seratonin giving us the 'feel good' factor we need in today's stress-filled world. Most nuts contain high quantities of carbohydrates and oils and should be eaten in moderation. Nut allergies have become more common in the past few years and can cause severe even fatal symptoms in some people. If there is any reason to suspect you have an allergy to nuts, have a test done. Many processed foods have traces of nuts and should be avoided if you have any form of nut allergy.

Composition of hazelnuts per 100g.

Nutrient	Unit	Raw
Water	g.	5.31
Energy	calories	628
Protein	g.	14.95
Lipid (fat)	g.	60.75
Fibre	g.	9.7

Nutrient		Unit	Raw
Sugars (total)		g.	4.34
Minerals:	Calcium	mg.	114
	Iron	mg.	4.70
Vitamins:	Vitamin A	mcg.	1
	Vitamin B1	mg.	0.643
	Vitamin B2	mg.	0.113
	Vitamin B6	mg.	0.563
	Vitamin C	mg.	6.3
	Vitamin E	mg.	15.03
	Niacin	mg.	1.800
	Folate	mcg.	113
	Pantothenic Acid	mg.	0.918

Sweet Corn ~ Properties

Sweet corn is nutritious and should be eaten as fresh as possible. Once removed from the stalk, the sugars quickly convert to starch. It is a good source of vitamin A , B1, C and dietary fibre. A reasonably high folate content makes it especially good for rebuilding red blood cells.

Composition of sweet corn per 100g.

Nutrient		Unit	Raw	Cooked
Water		g.	75.96	69.57
Energy		calories	86	108
Protein		g.	3.22	3.32
Lipid (fat)		g.	1.18	1.28
Fibre		g.	2.7	2.8
Sugars (total)		g.	3.22	3.17
Minerals:	Calcium	mg.	2	2
	Iron	mg.	0.52	0.61
Vitamins:	Vitamin A	mcg.	10	13
	Vitamin B1	mg.	0.200	0.215
	Vitamin B2	mg.	0.060	0.072
	Vitamin B6	mg.	0.055	0.060
	Vitamin C	mg.	6.8	6.2
	Vitamin E	mg.	0.07	0.09
	Niacin	mg.	1.700	1.614
	Folate	mcg.	46	46
	Pantothenic Acid	mg.	0.760	0.878

Vitamin B2 ~ Mushrooms, Salsify, Spinach, Watercress

Mushroom ~ Properties

Mushrooms are a good source of minerals and vitamins. They are not just a tasty addition to a meal, they also have plenty of nutrients. Mushrooms have been found to have anti-cancer properties and can help with many medical conditions, from menopausal problems to immune system deficiencies. During my years in France, I got to know many different edible varieties and I would hazard a guess that the people of France owe much of their good health to these delightful fungi. They are relatively high in protein and fibre, low in fat and they contain a range of vitamins...lots of great reasons to grow your own.

Composition of mushrooms per 100g.

Nutrient		Unit	Raw	Stir Fried
Water		g.	92.43	91.10
Energy		calories	22	26
Protein		g.	3.09	3.58
Lipid (fat)		g.	0.34	0.33
Fibre		g.	1.0	1.8
Sugars (total)		g.	1.65	0
Minerals:	Calcium	mg.	3	4
	Iron	mg.	0.50	0.25
Vitamins:	Vitamin A	mcg.	0	0
	Vitamin B1	mg.	0.081	0.096
	Vitamin B2	mg.	0.402	0.463
	Vitamin B6	mg.	0.104	0.042
	Vitamin C	mg.	2.1	0
	Vitamin E	mg.	0.01	0
	Niacin	mg.	3.607	3.987
	Folate	mcg.	16	20
	Pantothenic Acid	mg.	1.497	1.450

Salsify ~ Properties

Salsify is a good source of dietary fibre and contains no cholesterol or fat. A highly nutritious root vegetable, salsify is not commonly grown and is not often available in supermarkets. It is, however, worth growing for its nutritional value and the roots will stay healthy in the ground well into the winter months. The leaves are also edible and can be added raw to the salad bowl.

Composition of salsify per 100g.

Nutrient		Unit	Cooked
Water		g.	81.00
Energy		calories	68
Protein		g.	2.73
Lipid (fat)		g.	0.17
Fibre		g.	3.1
Sugars (total)		g.	2.90
Minerals:	Calcium	mg.	47
	Iron	mg.	0.55
Vitamins:	Vitamin A	mcg.	0
	Vitamin B1	mg.	0.056
	Vitamin B2	mg.	0.173
	Vitamin B6	mg.	0.218
	Vitamin C	mg.	4.6
	Vitamin E	mg.	0.19
	Niacin	mg.	0.392
	Folate	mcg.	15
	Pantothenic Acid	mg.	0.588

Spinach ~ Properties

Spinach has always been thought of as being the best form of iron in vegetable form for the human body. However, research has shown that the iron available in spinach is not easily absorbed by the body. Spinach contains B vitamins and a considerable amount of vitamin C. Overcooking reduces the available vitamins so spinach should be eaten raw or lightly cooked.

Composition of spinach per 100g.

Nutrient		Unit	Raw	Cooked
Water		g.	91.40	91.21
Energy		calories	23	23
Protein		g.	2.86	2.97
Lipid (fat)		g.	0.39	0.26
Fibre		g.	2.2	2.4
Sugars (total)		g.	0.42	0.43
Minerals:	Calcium	mg.	99	136
	Iron	mg.	2.71	3.57
Vitamins:	Vitamin A	mcg.	469	524
	Vitamin B1	mg.	0.078	0.095
	Vitamin B2	mg.	0.189	0.236

Nutrient		Unit	Raw	Cooked
Vitamin B6		mg.	0.195	0.242
Vitamin C		mg.	28.1	9.8
Vitamin E		mg.	2.03	2.08
Niacin		mg.	0.724	0.490
Folate		mcg.	194	146
Pantothenic Acid		mg.	0.065	0.145

Watercress ~ Properties

Watercress has been used in medicinal preparations since the 1st century. It was always thought to grow only in clear, running water but it will grow in any suitably moist condition in almost any moderate climate. Watercress is high in B vitamins and is a good source of vitamin C. As with all herbs, it should not be taken in very large doses. Don't plant watercress near sheep or cattle as the droppings from the animals can infect the plant with a deadly parasite.

Composition of watercress per 100g.

Nutrient		Unit	Raw
Water		g.	95.11
Energy		calories	11
Protein		g.	2.30
Lipid (fat)		g.	0.10
Fibre		g.	3.1
Sugars (total)		g.	0.5
Minerals:	Calcium	mg.	120
	Iron	mg.	0.20
Vitamins:	Vitamin A	mcg.	235
	Vitamin B1	mg.	0.090
	Vitamin B2	mg.	0.120
	Vitamin B6	mg.	0.129
	Vitamin C	mg.	43
	Vitamin E	mg.	0.07
	Niacin	mg.	0.200
	Folate	mcg.	9
	Pantothenic Acid	mg.	0.310

Vitamin B6 ~ Cabbage, Celeriac, Onions, Potatoes

Cabbage ~ Properties

Cabbage is high in vitamin C, B vitamins and has many other nutritional qualities. The purity of the vegetable has kept humankind healthy for centuries. With low calories, low fat and high vitamin content, cabbage should be part of our everyday diet. Preserved, fermented cabbage (sauerkraut) is an excellent source of vitamin K. The dark coloured varieties have a high beta-carotene content which helps the body produce vitamin A.

Composition of cabbage per 100g.

Nutrient		Unit	Raw	Cooked
Water		g.	92.15	92
Energy		calories	24	24
Protein		g.	1.44	1.80
Lipid (fat)		g.	0.12	0.09
Fibre		g.	2.3	2.8
Sugars (total)		g.	3.58	No data
Minerals:	Calcium	mg.	47	30
	Iron	mg.	.59	.38
Vitamins:	Vitamin A	mcg.	9	44
	Vitamin B1	mg.	0.050	0.051
	Vitamin B2	mg.	0.040	0.020
	Vitamin B6	mg.	0.096	0.152
	Vitamin C	mg.	32.2	17
	Vitamin E	mg.	0.15	No data
	Niacin	mg.	0.300	0.024
	Folate	mcg.	43	46
	Pantothenic Acid	mg.	0.140	0.159

Celeriac ~ Properties

Celeriac is a member of the celery family but hasn't been commonly grown in home vegetable plots in recent years. It used to be a very popular root vegetable. With a high vitamin content, it is low in fat and is a good source of dietary fibre. Celeriac can be added to cooked meals for added flavour or eaten raw, grated in salad.

Composition of celeriac per 100g.

Nutrient	Unit	Raw	Cooked
Water	g.	88.00	92.30
Energy	calories	42	27

Nutrient		Unit	Raw	Cooked
Protein		g.	1.50	0.96
Lipid (fat)		g.	0.30	0.19
Fibre		g.	1.8	1.2
Sugars (total)		g.	1.60	0
Minerals:	Calcium	mg.	43	26
	Iron	mg.	0.70	0.43
Vitamins:	Vitamin A	mcg.	0	0
	Vitamin B1	mg.	0.050	0.027
	Vitamin B2	mg.	0.060	0.037
	Vitamin B6	mg.	0.165	0.101
	Vitamin C	mg.	8.0	3.6
	Vitamin E	mg.	0.36	0
	Niacin	mg.	0.700	0.427
	Folate	mcg.	8	3
	Pantothenic Acid	mg.	0.352	0.203

Onion ~ Properties

Onions have been proved to balance insulin levels, therefore reducing blood sugar. They are one of the few vegetables that significantly reduce the risk of heart disease through lowering cholesterol and high blood pressure. Onions are a good source of B vitamins and vitamin C, as well as dietary fibre. No kitchen should be without them.

Composition of onions per 100g.

Nutrient		Unit	Raw	Cooked
Water		g.	88.54	87.86
Energy		calories	42	44
Protein		g.	0.92	1.36
Lipid (fat)		g.	0.08	0.19
Fibre		g.	1.4	1.4
Sugars (total)		g.	4.28	4.53
Minerals:	Calcium	mg.	22	22
	Iron	mg.	0.19	0.24
Vitamins:	Vitamin A	mcg.	0	0
	Vitamin B1	mg.	0.048	0.042
	Vitamin B2	mg.	0.025	0.023
	Vitamin B6	mg.	0.147	0.129
	Vitamin C	mg.	6.4	5.2

Nutrient	Unit	Raw	Cooked
Vitamin E	mg.	0.02	0.02
Niacin	mg.	0.083	0.165
Folate	mcg.	19	15
Pantothenic Acid	mg.	0.122	0.113

Potato ~ Properties

Potatoes are nutritious and nourishing and form a big part of the western diet. They are a valuable source of vitamin C, the B vitamins, carbohydrates and minerals. Over the last couple of centuries, the potato has been used as a medicinal food for various ailments including digestive problems. It is also said to be a good cure for dry skin and sores (mix grated raw potato with a little olive oil and apply to affected area).

Composition of potatoes per 100g.

Nutrient		Unit	Boiled – no salt or skin	Mashed with milk & marg.
Water		g.	77.46	75.24
Energy		calories	86	113
Protein		g.	1.71	2.00
Lipid (fat)		g.	0.10	4.19
Fibre		g.	1.8	1.5
Sugars (total)		g.	0.085	1.44
Minerals:	Calcium	mg.	8	22
	Iron	mg.	0.31	0.26
Vitamins:	Vitamin A	mcg.	0	41
	Vitamin B1	mg.	0.098	0.092
	Vitamin B2	mg.	0.019	0.044
	Vitamin B6	mg.	0.269	0.247
	Vitamin C	mg.	7.4	10.5
	Vitamin E	mg.	0.01	0.42
	Niacin	mg.	1.312	1.176
	Folate	mcg.	9	9
	Pantothenic Acid	mg.	.0.509	0.474

Vitamin C ~ Blackcurrants, Peppers, Strawberries, Tomato

Blackcurrant ~ Properties

Blackcurrants have four times the vitamin C content of oranges and are a lot less acidic. They are rich in natural antioxidants and are one of the most popular edible fruits across the globe. Almost all of the commercial blackcurrant production in the UK goes to making blackcurrant juice. They are used to flavour many products from medicine to ice cream.

Composition of blackcurrants per 100g.

Nutrient		Unit	Raw
Water		g.	81.96
Energy		calories	63
Protein		g.	1.40
Lipid (fat)		g.	0.41
Nutrient		Unit	Raw
Fibre		g.	5.8
Sugars (total)		g.	7.8
Minerals:	Calcium	mg.	55
	Iron	mg.	1.54
Vitamins:	Vitamin A	mcg.	12
	Vitamin B1	mg.	0.050
	Vitamin B2	mg.	0.050
	Vitamin B6	mg.	0.066
	Vitamin C	mg.	181.0
	Vitamin E	mg.	1.0
	Niacin	mg.	0.300
	Folate	mcg.	No data
	Pantothenic Acid	mg.	0.398

Pepper ~ Properties

Peppers are very high in vitamins C and A – higher than most other fruits and vegetables. The beta-carotene and lycopene content, especially in mature red fruits, means the pepper has antioxidant properties and has been proven to act on free radicals in the human body. Red peppers contain twice the amount of vitamin C as green peppers. Peppers help the body absorb iron and calcium and are a beneficial food for those convalescing after an operation or illness. They are easy to grow, easy to cook and above all, they provide huge quantities of vitamins and minerals for your family. Peppers are very effective in a weight loss programme as they have a high water content and can be eaten raw. Chilli peppers are the spicy variety of pepper and should be eaten in moderation by those with a delicate stomach or digestive system. Otherwise there is no limit to the amount of peppers you can add to your diet.

Composition of sweet green peppers per 100g.

Nutrient		Unit	Raw	Cooked
Water		g.	93.89	82.65
Energy		calories	20	127
Protein		g.	0.86	0.78
Lipid (fat)		g.	0.17	11.85
Fibre		g.	1.7	1.8
Sugars (total)		g.	2.40	2.17
Minerals:	Calcium	mg.	10	8
	Iron	mg.	0.34	0.30
Vitamins:	Vitamin A	mcg.	18	14
	Vitamin B1	mg.	0.057	0.042
	Vitamin B2	mg.	0.028	0.048
	Vitamin C	mg.	80.4	177.0
	Vitamin E	mg.	0.37	1.40
	Niacin	mg.	0.480	0.582
	Folate	mcg.	151	2
	Pantothenic Acid	mg.	0.099	0.111

Composition of hot Chilli peppers per 100g.

Nutrient		Unit	Red, raw	Green, raw
Water		g.	88.02	87.74
Energy		calories	40	40
Protein		g.	1.87	2.00
Lipid (fat)		g.	0.44	0.20
Fibre		g.	1.5	1.5
Sugars (total)		g.	5.30	5.10
Minerals:	Calcium	mg.	14	18
	Iron	mg.	1.03	1.20
Vitamins:	Vitamin A	mcg.	48	59
	Vitamin B1	mg.	0.072	0.090
	Vitamin B2	mg.	0.086	0.090
	Vitamin B6	mg.	0.506	0.278
	Vitamin C	mg.	143.7	242.5
	Vitamin E	mg.	0.69	0.69

Nutrient		Unit	Red, raw	Green, raw
	Niacin	mg.	1.244	0.950
	Folate	mcg.	23	23
	Pantothenic Acid	mg.	0.201	0.061

Strawberry ~ Properties

Strawberries, like all berries, are strong antioxidants and help protect the body against various cell-damaging diseases, including some forms of cancer. They contain phenol, which makes them anti-inflammatory, helping to alleviate symptoms of rheumatoid arthritis, asthma and other illnesses. Strawberries are high in vitamin C content and dietary fibre.

Composition of strawberries per 100g.

Nutrient		Unit	Raw
Water		g.	90.95
Energy		calories	32
Protein		g.	0.67
Lipid (fat)		g.	0.30
Fibre		g.	2.0
Sugars (total)		g.	4.66
Minerals:	Calcium	mg.	16
	Iron	mg.	0.42
Vitamins:	Vitamin A	mcg.	1
	Vitamin B1	mg.	0.024
	Vitamin B2	mg.	0.022
	Vitamin B6	mg.	0.078
	Vitamin C	mg.	58.8
	Vitamin E	mg.	0.29
	Niacin	mg.	0.386
	Folate	mcg.	24
	Pantothenic Acid	mg.	0.125

Tomato ~ Properties

Tomatoes are a good source of vitamin C and they also retain vitamin C after cooking which many fruits and vegetables do not. Research shows that people with a higher intake of tomatoes in their diet are at a lower risk of developing certain cancers. Tomatoes are low in sodium and high in minerals. They are also rich in vitamin A and low in calories. A regular tomato measuring approximately 2" across will weigh around 70 grams.

Thank you for buying this book. If you would like to receive any further information about our product list, please return this card after filling in your areas of interest.

Title of this book..

If purchased : Retailer's name.............................. Town..............

☐ Health and Nutrition   ☐ Philosophy & Spirituality

☐ Indigenous Cultures   ☐ Psychology & Psychotherapy

☐ Occult & Divination   ☐ Women's Interest

☐ Personal Growth   ☐ Other

Name...

Address..

....

....

DEEP BOOKS LTD
UNIT 3 GOOSE GREEN TRADING ESTATE
47 EAST DULWICH ROAD
LONDON
SE22 9BN
UK

Composition of tomatoes per 100g.

Nutrient		Unit	Raw	Cooked
Water		g.	94.50	94.34
Energy		calories	18	18
Protein		g.	0.88	0.95
Lipid (fat)		g.	0.20	0.11
Fibre		g.	1.2	0.7
Sugars (total)		g.	2.63	2.49
Minerals:	Calcium	mg.	10	11
	Iron	mg.	0.27	0.68
Vitamins:	Vitamin A	mcg.	42	24
	Vitamin B1	mg.	0.037	0.036
	Vitamin B2	mg.	0.019	0.022
	Vitamin B6	mg.	0.080	0.079
	Vitamin C	mg.	12.7	22.8
	Vitamin E	mg.	0.54	0.56
	Niacin	mg.	0.594	0.532
	Folate	mcg.	15	13
	Pantothenic Acid	mg.	0.089	0.129

Vitamin E ~ Asparagus, Dandelion greens, Raspberries, Sunflower seeds

Asparagus ~ Properties

Asparagus is known to have many medicinal properties and sufferers of kidney problems, water retention or those carrying extra weight will do well to include a regular serving of asparagus in their diet. It can be eaten raw or cooked. Asparagus is very low in calories and is also believed to help certain heart conditions. The water in which we cook asparagus can be used to make a healthy drink.

Composition of asparagus per 100g.

Nutrient		Unit	Raw	Cooked
Water		g.	93.22	92.63
Energy		calories	20	22
Protein		g.	2.20	2.40
Lipid (fat)		g.	0.12	0.22
Fibre		g.	2.1	2.0
Sugars (total)		g.	1.88	1.30
Minerals:	Calcium	mg.	24	23

Nutrient		Unit	Raw	Cooked
	Iron	mg.	2.14	0.91
Vitamins:	Vitamin A	mcg.	38	50
	Vitamin B1	mg.	0.143	0.162
	Vitamin B2	mg.	0.141	0.139
	Vitamin B6	mg.	0.091	0.079
	Vitamin C	mg.	5.6	7.7
	Vitamin E	mg.	1.13	1.50
	Niacin	mg.	0.978	1.084
	Folate	mcg.	52	149
	Pantothenic Acid	mg.	.0.274	0.225

Dandelion Green ~ Properties

Dandelions are high in vitamins A , E and C, and also contain an easy to digest form of iron. They are a natural diuretic and a glass or two of dandelion tea will relieve that bloated feeling when retaining too much water. Dandelion leaf is reported to be very effective in treating anaemia due to its high vitamin B complex content.

Composition of dandelion greens per 55g.

Nutrient		Unit	Raw	% RDA
Water		%	86	–
Energy		calories	24.7	1%
Protein		g.	1.5	3%
Lipid (fat)		g.	0.4	1%
Fibre		g.	2	8%
Sugars (total)		g.	2	–
Minerals:	Calcium	mg.	–	10%
	Iron	mg.	–	9%
Vitamins:	Vitamin A	mcg.	–	54%
	Vitamin B1	mg.	0.1	7%
	Vitamin B2	mg.	0.1	8%
	Vitamin B6	mg.	0.1	7%
	Vitamin C	mg.	19.3	32%
	Vitamin E	mg.	2.6	9%
	Niacin	mg.	0.4	2%
	Folate	mcg.	14.9	4%
	Pantothenic Acid	mg.	0.0	0%

Raspberry ~ Properties

A good source of vitamins and dietary fibre, raspberries also have 50% more antioxidants than strawberries and play a great part in protecting the body against cell damaging diseases. A few raspberries in the diet count towards the vitamins, fibre and fruit we need on a daily basis. Frozen raspberries contain about half the vitamin C content of fresh raspberries.

Composition of raspberries per 100g.

Nutrient		Unit	Raw
Water		g.	85.75
Energy		calories	52
Protein		g.	1.20
Lipid (fat)		g.	0.65
Fibre		g.	6.5
Sugars (total)		g.	4.42
Minerals:	Calcium	mg.	25
	Iron	mg.	0.69
Vitamins:	Vitamin A	mcg.	2
	Vitamin B1	mg.	0.032
	Vitamin B2	mg.	0.038
	Vitamin B6	mg.	0.055
	Vitamin C	mg.	26.2
	Vitamin E	mg.	0.87
	Niacin	mg.	0.598
	Folate	mcg.	21
	Pantothenic Acid	mg.	0.329

Sunflower Seed ~ Properties

Sunflower seeds are high in mineral and vitamin content. The flower petals are poisonous and should not be eaten under any circumstances. If you wish to add bright colour to your salad recipes, you can use marigolds or other edible plants but NEVER sunflowers. The seeds are the part you eat, which means you get to enjoy the majestic flowers right through the summer growing season and then harvest the seeds when the plant has finished blooming. Sunflower seeds can contain up to 50% unsaturated oil and are high in nutrients for animals and humans.

Composition of sunflower seeds per 100g.

Nutrient	Unit	Dry roasted no salt	Oil roasted with salt
Water	g.	1.20	1.54
Energy	calories	582	592

Nutrient		Unit	Dry roasted no salt	Oil roasted with salt
Protein		g.	19.33	20.06
Lipid (fat)		g.	49.80	51.30
Fibre		g.	11.1	10.6
Sugars (total)		g.	2.73	3.11
Minerals:	Calcium	mg.	70	87
	Iron	mg.	3.80	4.28
Vitamins:	Vitamin A	mcg.	0	9
	Vitamin B1	mg.	0.106	0.320
	Vitamin B2	mg.	0.246	0.280
	Vitamin B6	mg.	0.804	0.792
	Vitamin C	mg.	1.4	1.1
	Vitamin E	mg.	26.10	36.33
	Niacin	mg.	7.042	4.130
	Folate	mcg.	237	234
	Pantothenic Acid	mg.	7.042	6.942

Folate ~ Beetroot, Green beans, Parsley, Turnip greens

Beetroot ~ Properties
Beet or beetroot is an excellent source of folate, vitamin C and dietary fibre. Beetroot, often pickled or consumed as a soup, is said to be a main factor in longevity, as it was regularly consumed by the well-known Russian centenarians. The rich pigment is a powerful agent in fighting free radicals. Although traditionally pickled, beets can be enjoyed in many different ways, including steamed or grated raw in salads.

Composition of beetroot per 100g.

Nutrient		Unit	Cooked
Water		g.	87.06
Energy		calories	44
Protein		g.	1.68
Lipid (fat)		g.	0.18
Fibre		g.	2.0
Sugars (total)		g.	7.96
Minerals:	Calcium	mg.	16
	Iron	mg.	0.79
Vitamins:	Vitamin A	mcg.	2
	Vitamin B1	mg.	0.027

Nutrient		Unit	Cooked
	Vitamin B2	mg.	0.040
	Vitamin B6	mg.	0.067
	Vitamin C	mg.	3.6
	Vitamin E	mg.	0.04
	Niacin	mg.	0.331
	Folate	mcg.	80
	Pantothenic Acid	mg.	0.145

Green Bean ~ Properties

Green beans are a good source of calcium and vitamins A and C, as well as folate. They should always be cooked before eating. Green beans (also known as flageolets, snap beans, bush beans and string beans) aid digestion and are safe to eat every day. The water they are cooked or steamed in will contain iron and should be used in gravy or sauces if possible. Beans are high in protein and dietary fibre.

Composition of green beans per 100g.

Nutrient		Unit	Cooked
Water		g.	89.22
Energy		calories	35
Protein		g.	1.89
Lipid (fat)		g.	0.28
Fibre		g.	3.2
Sugars (total)		g.	1.55
Minerals:	Calcium	mg.	44
	Iron	mg.	0.65
Vitamins:	Vitamin A	mcg.	35
	Vitamin B1	mg.	0.074
	Vitamin B2	mg.	0.097
	Vitamin B6	mg.	0.056
	Vitamin C	mg.	9.7
	Vitamin E	mg.	0.45
	Niacin	mg.	0.614
	Folate	mcg.	33
	Pantothenic Acid	mg.	0.074

Parsley ~ Properties

Parsley is relatively high in vitamins A and C and many of the B vitamins including B3 (niacin). It contains minerals that are easily absorbed, and although parsley has traditionally been used as a garnish, it is now being recognised as a valuable herb and is included in many recipes.

Composition of parsley per 100g.

Nutrient		Unit	Raw	Dried
Water		g.	87.71	9.02
Energy		calories	36	276
Protein		g.	2.97	22.42
Lipid (fat)		g.	0.79	4.43
Fibre		g.	3.3	30.4
Sugars (total)		g.	0.85	7.27
Minerals:	Calcium	mg.	138	1468
	Iron	mg.	6.20	97.86
Vitamins:	Vitamin A	mcg.	421	509
	Vitamin B1	mg.	0.086	0.172
	Vitamin B2	mg.	0.098	1.230
	Vitamin B6	mg.	0.090	1.002
	Vitamin C	mg.	133.0	122.0
	Vitamin E	mg.	0.75	6.91
	Niacin	mg.	1.313	7.929
	Folate	mcg.	152	180
	Pantothenic Acid	mg.	0.400	No data

Turnip Green ~ Properties

Turnip greens are rich in folate, vitamin C, minerals, and dietary fibre. They contain goitrogens and shouldn't be eaten by individuals with untreated thyroid problems.

Composition of turnip greens per 100g.

Nutrient		Unit	Cooked
Water		g.	93.20
Energy		calories	20
Protein		g.	1.14
Lipid (fat)		g.	0.23
Fibre		g.	3.5
Sugars (total)		g.	0.53
Minerals:	Calcium	mg.	137
	Iron	mg.	0.80
Vitamins:	Vitamin A	mcg.	381
	Vitamin B1	mg.	0.045
	Vitamin B2	mg.	0.072

Nutrient	Unit	Cooked
Vitamin B6	mg.	0.180
Vitamin C	mg.	27.4
Vitamin E	mg.	1.88
Niacin	mg.	0.411
Folate	mcg.	118
Pantothenic Acid	mg.	0.274

Niacin ~ Aubergine (Eggplant), Courgette (Zucchini), Fennel bulb, Peas

Aubergine ~ Properties

The deep purple colour of aubergine, or eggplant, is due to pigments with antioxidant properties. These pigments help control free radicals so aubergines may have anti-cancer properties. They are high in fibre and there have been reports suggesting extracts of aubergine can help lower blood cholesterol.

Composition of aubergine per 100g.

Nutrient		Unit	Cooked
Water		g.	89.67
Energy		calories	35
Protein		g.	0.83
Lipid (fat)		g.	0.23
Fibre		g.	2.5
Sugars (total)		g.	3.20
Minerals:	Calcium	mg.	6
	Iron	mg.	0.25
Vitamins:	Vitamin A	mcg.	2
	Vitamin B1	mg.	0.076
	Vitamin B2	mg.	0.020
	Vitamin B6	mg.	0.086
	Vitamin C	mg.	1.3
	Vitamin E	mg.	0.41
	Niacin	mg.	0.600
	Folate	mcg.	14
	Pantothenic Acid	mg.	0.075

Courgette ~ Properties

Courgettes (zucchini) are immature marrows but so much tastier. They are part of the gourd family and provide a good source of vitamins. Eat them young and unpeeled for maximum effect. The seeds are also beneficial as they contain natural chemicals that help to control enlargement of the prostate gland – a very common condition in men over 50.

When courgette plants take hold they tend to be prolific so you may have to find creative ways to use them. In addition to being a stand-alone veggie, part of a multi-veg casserole, or raw in a salad, they can even be baked into a delicious bread.

Composition of courgettes per 100g.

Nutrient		Unit	Cooked
Water		g.	94.74
Energy		calories	16
Protein		g.	0.64
Lipid (fat)		g.	0.05
Fibre		g.	1.4
Sugars (total)		g.	1.69
Minerals:	Calcium	mg.	13
	Iron	mg.	0.35
Vitamins:	Vitamin A	mcg.	56
	Vitamin B1	mg.	0.041
	Vitamin B2	mg.	0.041
	Vitamin B6	mg.	0.078
	Vitamin C	mg.	4.6
	Vitamin E	mg.	0.12
	Niacin	mg.	0.428
	Folate	mcg.	17
	Pantothenic Acid	mg.	0.114

Fennel Bulb ~ Properties

Fennel has a calming effect on the body. It helps to relieve indigestion and to digest fatty or oily foods. Fennel also helps alleviate cold and flu symptoms. Its strong aniseed odour and flavour make it ideal for flavouring drinks, sweets and medicines, and for adding to perfume and scented soaps. It is a good source of dietary fibre and makes a wonderful addition to any meal.

Composition of fennel bulb per 100g.

Nutrient	Unit	Raw
Water	g.	90.21
Energy	calories	31
Protein	g.	1.24
Lipid (fat)	g.	0.20
Fibre	g.	3.1

Nutrient		Unit	Raw
Sugars (total)		g.	No data
Minerals:	Calcium	mg.	49
	Iron	mg.	0.73
Vitamins:	Vitamin A	mcg.	7
	Vitamin B1	mg.	0.010
	Vitamin B2	mg.	0.032
	Vitamin B6	mg.	0.047
	Vitamin C	mg.	12.0
	Vitamin E	mg.	No data
	Niacin	mg.	0.640
	Folate	mcg.	27
	Pantothenic Acid	mg.	0.232

Pea ~ Properties

Peas are a good source of vitamins, including A and C, which are strong antioxidants that help to neutralise free radicals. Peas are also a protein rich vegetable. Niacin (B3) is one of the B vitamins present in peas and helps the body absorb iron. Peas are also said to reduce the risk of some age-related conditions.

Composition of peas per 100g.

Nutrient		Unit	Raw	Cooked
Water		g.	78.86	77.87
Energy		calories	81	84
Protein		g.	5.42	5.36
Lipid (fat)		g.	0.40	0.22
Fibre		g.	5.1	5.5
Sugars (total)		g.	5.67	5.93
Minerals:	Calcium	mg.	25	27
	Iron	mg.	1.47	1.54
Vitamins:	Vitamin A	mcg.	765	40
	Vitamin B1	mg.	0.266	0.259
	Vitamin B2	mg.	0.132	0.149
	Vitamin B6	mg.	0.169	0.216
	Vitamin C	mg.	40.0	14.2
	Vitamin E	mg.	0.13	0.14
	Niacin	mg.	2.090	2.021
	Folate	mcg.	65	63
	Pantothenic Acid	mg.	0.104	0.153

P antothenic Acid ~ Broccoli, Cauliflower, Chicory, Parsnip

Broccoli ~ Properties

Broccoli is considered to be a 'super food' and is gaining in popularity, although it is not much different than most other brassicas, such as cauliflower and cabbage. Broccoli is packed with vitamins and minerals, and if you choose the purple sprouting variety, it contains even more antioxidants than regular green varieties.

Composition of broccoli per 100g.

Nutrient		Unit	Cooked
Water		g.	89.25
Energy		calories	35
Protein		g.	2.38
Lipid (fat)		g.	0.41
Fibre		g.	3.3
Sugars (total)		g.	1.39
Minerals:	Calcium	mg.	40
	Iron	mg.	0.67
Vitamins:	Vitamin A	mcg.	77
	Vitamin B1	mg.	0.063
	Vitamin B2	mg.	0.123
	Vitamin B6	mg.	0.200
	Vitamin C	mg.	64.9
	Vitamin E	mg.	1.45
	Niacin	mg.	0.553
	Folate	mcg.	108
	Pantothenic Acid	mg.	0.616

Cauliflower ~ Properties

Cauliflower, along with other brassicas, helps reduce the risk of cancer. Because compounds in brassicas help the liver neutralise toxins efficiently, they are good detox vegetables. Cauliflower is also rich in vitamin C, folate and dietary fibre.

Composition of cauliflower per 100g.

Nutrient	Unit	Cooked
Water	g.	93.0
Energy	calories	23
Protein	g.	1.84
Lipid (fat)	g.	0.45
Fibre	g.	2.7

Nutrient		Unit	Cooked
Sugars (total)		g.	1.41
Minerals:	Calcium	mg.	16
	Iron	mg.	0.33
Vitamins:	Vitamin A	mcg.	1
	Vitamin B1	mg.	0.042
	Vitamin B2	mg.	0.052
	Vitamin B6	mg.	0.173
	Vitamin C	mg.	44.3
	Vitamin E	mg.	0.07
	Niacin	mg.	0.410
	Folate	mcg.	44
	Pantothenic Acid	mg.	0.508

Chicory ~ Properties

Chicory is usually grown as a salad crop but the plant is often 'forced' in dark conditions to create the white vegetable the French eat as 'endive'. Chicory is high in mineral and vitamin content and is considered to be a good all round tonic. It was traditionally used to treat liver complaints.

Composition of chicory and endive per 100g.

Nutrient		Unit	Chicory leaves	Endive
Water		%	92.0	93.79
Energy		calories	23	17
Protein		g.	1.70	1.25
Lipid (fat)		g.	0.30	0.20
Fibre		g.	4.0	3.1
Sugars (total)		g.	0.70	0.25
Minerals:	Calcium	mg.	100	52
	Iron	mg.	0.90	0.83
Vitamins:	Vitamin A	mcg.	286	108
	Vitamin B1	mg.	0.060	0.080
	Vitamin B2	mg.	0.100	0.075
	Vitamin B6	mg.	0.105	0.020
	Vitamin C	mg.	24.0	6.5
	Vitamin E	mg.	2.26	0.44
	Niacin	mg.	0.500	0.400
	Folate	mcg.	110	142
	Pantothenic Acid	mg.	1.159	0.900

Parsnip ~ Properties

Parsnips are closely related to the carrot but are richer in minerals and vitamins. They are also rich in potassium and dietary fibre and are a wonderful wholesome winter vegetable. Take extra care if collecting wild parsnips as the plant closely resembles the deadly poison, hemlock.

Composition of parsnips per 100g.

Nutrient		Unit	Cooked
Water		g.	80.24
Energy		calories	71
Protein		g.	1.32
Lipid (fat)		g.	0.30
Fibre		g.	3.6
Sugars (total)		g.	4.80
Minerals:	Calcium	mg.	37
	Iron	mg.	0.58
Vitamins:	Vitamin A	mcg.	0
	Vitamin B1	mg.	0.083
	Vitamin B2	mg.	0.051
	Vitamin B6	mg.	0.093
	Vitamin C	mg.	13.0
	Vitamin E	mg.	1.00
	Niacin	mg.	0.724
	Folate	mcg.	58
	Pantothenic Acid	mg.	0.588

Chapter Four

Growing Plants Rich in Vitamin A

Carrots, Cos Lettuce (Romaine), Kale, Pumpkin

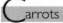Carrots

History

The carrot is thought to have been cultivated 5000 years ago in many different colours including purple, red, yellow and black varieties. The bright orange variety we know today was developed in Holland when the Dutch crossed a red and yellow variety in the 16th century. There are many references to carrot-like vegetables over the centuries; however the carrot is closely related to the parsnip, and some accounts are unclear as to which root vegetable was being referenced. The Romans brought garden carrots with them when they invaded Britain in the second century AD. Greeks used carrots as an aphrodisiac to increase ardour in both men and women.

Growing Methods

Choosing your carrots ~ Although we tend to buy only orange carrots to grow in our gardens, there are many varieties we can experiment with. Carrots are a taproot vegetable and they come in various shapes and sizes. There are yellow, red and purple varieties readily available alongside the regular orange types in garden centres and global seed suppliers. If you have plenty of depth to your soil, a long carrot will do well, but if your good soil tends to be shallow, go for a shorter variety.

Prepare the site ~ The soil should be fairly light and needs to be prepared thoroughly to ensure a good crop of carrots. Work to about 12 in. (30 cm.) deep and remove all weeds, stones and other debris. Carrots are a taproot vegetable and need a clean, clear passage to develop fully.

If the ground is too heavy, dig in a little sand. The cleaner and well-drained the soil, the more cylindrical your carrots will be. They also will be tastier and more usable. Although you can use mis-shaped carrots, they aren't as easy to prepare and cook as those with a good cylindrical shape.

Position ~ Carrots will tolerate a little shade and can be planted in short lines in your herb garden or flower beds if space is hard to find. They like sunlight and will benefit from a bright growing area even if a little shady at times. Carrots grown in full sun tend to need more attention to watering. They need warmth to fully develop, and planting in particularly cold spots or cross winds should be avoided if possible.

Sowing carrots ~ Cloches may be used, but carefully. Remove the cloche during the day as much as possible to avoid moss and stagnant soil particles developing. Carrots like fresh air. They aren't a tropical vegetable so will not grow well in humid or very hot environments.

When you have your seeds and your ground is prepared, check the dates on your seed packets for advice as to when you should be sowing in your area. Some varieties can be planted earlier than others.

Don't plant in waterlogged or frozen ground. The seeds just won't germinate. Prepare your plot and mark the ends of your rows. Carrots are notorious for long germination periods and marking rows helps to remember where you planted them. Gently cover the seed and water carefully.

Carrots are best planted in short rows. Sow your seeds in 60 cm. rows, **maximum**! There is a good reason for this. When your carrots start germinating – and they do take some time so a little patience is needed – they will need to be thinned out along each row.

Knowing what the newly sprouting carrot plant looks like is useful. Then you can pull the weeds without fear of pulling up your new carrot plants. As carrots take some time to germinate, there will inevitably be weeds that appear before the carrots do.

When the carrots are between 3 and 5 cm. tall, it's time to start thinning. Don't try and thin your carrots if the ground is very dry; water first if necessary. Then gently lift the baby plants out leaving one plant every centimetre and gently firm the soil around the remaining plants if they lift a little.

Keep weed-free and watered. In a couple of weeks when the carrots start to fill up the gaps and are around 5–8 cm. tall, thin them again, allowing 1–2 cm. per plant. You should be pulling very tiny carrots now. These small carrots are very nutritious and should be eaten. They can be rinsed and tossed into the salad bowl or even stir-fried.

The last thinning session takes place a few weeks later and you should allow around 3–5 cm. per carrot depending on the type. Allow more space for wider varieties. After the last thinning, keep the rows of carrots watered and free of weeds until they are fully grown.

After you have sown the first line of carrots, keep a note of the date and plant a new line every couple of weeks to ensure a constant supply of fully grown carrots and also small carrots, collected when you thin the lines.

Caring for your carrots ~ Carrots tend to be fairly hardy and should keep growing well if they have enough water and warmth throughout the growing season. They don't like to dry out and during long, dry periods, you should water every day.

Try to thin your carrots when it's raining to avoid the carrot fly. Another way to avoid pests and disease is to plant alongside onions. A row of onions next to a row of carrots helps prevent the carrot fly getting to the carrots and the onion fly getting to the onions.

Carrots can be left in the ground until the first frost; some varieties are frost resistant. I've pulled carrots out of snow-covered ground, although it isn't ideal. It's best to harvest your crop just before the first frost depending on the variety. Check your seed packets for regional advice. It's also a good idea to find out what other growers are doing in your area. Listen to advice from those gardeners who produce great vegetables.

Poly-tunnels and containers

Carrots thrive in outdoor conditions but if given enough depth of soil and enough light, there should be no reason why you can't grow them in a poly-tunnel or container. Containers must be deep, well-drained and the soil kept moist at all times. Containers tend to dry out very quickly.

Storing

Carrots store well throughout the winter if kept in a dry, dark place. Don't wash them before storing. As soon as carrots are washed they start to deteriorate and will not store well.

The best way to store carrots through the winter months is in a sack or barrel of dry sand kept in a dry, dark storeroom. Watch out for mice invasions though. Hang sacks from hooks in the ceiling, if possible or make sure the barrel is mouse-proof.

Carrots can be frozen or bottled (canned) and it's better to use younger vegetables for these methods. Slicing carrots and freezing on trays before bagging works well. Carrots and garden peas are a popular frozen vegetable in grocery stores but there's no reason why you can't produce your own.

Cos Lettuce

History

Cos, or romaine lettuce has been cultivated for around 5000 years and is probably one of the oldest cultivated lettuces known. It is thought to have originated in eastern Mediterranean areas and western Europe. Cos has been a popular vegetable in the Orient for many years and is considered to represent good luck in China. The milky liquid in the leaf stems has been used in herbal preparations since ancient times. It's thought that lettuce is a very easy vegetable to grow in the home garden, but in fact it needs a little extra care to ensure a healthy crop.

Growing Cos Lettuce

Choosing cos lettuce ~ Cos lettuce grows into a pointed head. Cos tends to be more resistant to bolting than most other lettuces, in other words, they don't run to seed so quickly in hot, dry weather. However they do need watering more regularly than most plants during dry periods.

The cos variety of lettuce is a particular type and it is unusual to find a choice of varieties. There may be a hybrid available in your local garden centre but check on results first as the growing conditions may need adjusting.

Prepare the site ~ Lettuce seed is very small and if sowing directly outside, the seedbed should be very well hoed and weeded. Remove all stones from the seed area. Lettuce will benefit from a fairly rich soil, and digging in well-rotted compost earlier in the year or the previous autumn is preferable.

Position ~ Although lettuce is a vegetable we tend to eat during summer months, it prefers a slightly cooler climate to grow well. So direct sunlight isn't particularly good for cos or any other lettuce. Cos is more resistant to the heat but still prefers a little shade during the hottest parts of the day. When lettuces are ready for transplanting, they can be popped in between small shrubs in the flower or herb bed. The shrubs will provide them with the shade they need and this also helps save space in the vegetable garden.

Sowing cos lettuce ~ Start your seeds in seed trays in a greenhouse, conservatory or even on a warm windowsill. Use an organic, all purpose seed compost and keep warm and watered until the plants are a few inches high.

Alternatively you could start the seed directly in the outside seedbed, but the seed won't germinate if there's a frost so, depending on your region, you may have to wait until May to sow seed outside.

To ensure a summer supply, start the seed inside as early as March or even February if you can keep the soil warm enough. Again this depends on your region. Check on the seed packet for suggested sowing times, or talk to local gardeners and find out what they do. As soon as the plants start to show themselves, you must protect against slugs and snails.

Even though lettuce seeds are small they tend to germinate well. With this in mind, it's advisable to plant just a very short line or a few seeds at a time, leaving 2–4 weeks between sowings. Then you have a constant supply. There is a limit to how much lettuce you can eat. I've made the mistake of sowing too many seeds and even my chickens grew tired of eating lettuce!

When the lettuces are a few inches high, and have a number of true leaves, it's time to thin them out. If the weather is still a bit cold at night, I replant the small lettuce plants in more trays or large pots and keep them in the greenhouse for an extra week or two. When transplanting always make sure they are well watered.

When the weather is warm enough, plant outside, either dotted around the garden or in rows, leaving about 8 in. (20 cm.) between plants and around 18 in. (45 cm.) between rows. The best time to transplant is in the morning if possible, and on a day when there is perhaps a light rain or at least a few clouds and not very hot sunshine.

Putting any small plants out in hot sunshine will cause them to wilt and could burn the leaves before they even get going. Sometimes it may be advisable to shade your young plants with a special shading sheet, available from most garden centres. Positioning well from the start is the best way. Make sure there is sufficient shade from the midday sun.

Caring for cos lettuce ~ The biggest enemy of the young lettuce plant is the slug. A slug can wipe out a whole row of lettuce in a very short time. You have to be vigilant even in the greenhouse. Use organic means of dealing with slug and snail problems, rather than putting chemicals in your soil.

Slugs and snails won't have any scruples, and will be delighted with the gift of freshly planted, young lettuces for them to eat. The fact that you've nurtured the baby plants for weeks is irrelevant to them.

There are a number of things snails and slugs really don't like. It takes a little organising but it's worth the effort. They don't like eggshells. Crush shells and lay them as thickly as possible around each lettuce. Don't leave any gaps.

Some gardeners swear by beer, for the pests that is. Sink a bowl of beer into the ground close to the lettuces and it attracts the slugs and snails to it. They fall in, get drunk and drown. This is okay if you don't mind dealing with a lot of dead slugs and snails every morning.

Placing a plastic circle around the plants and sprinkling salt right round is another deterrent. Make sure there are no gaps though. Those cunning slugs will find the loophole if there is one.

There are organic products that may help to prevent a slug attack as well. Check with your garden centre.

Apart from the pests, keep lettuces well watered, especially in long, dry periods. Once gone to seed, they become bitter and inedible. Also keep weeded and hoe round the plants gently from time to time.

Poly-tunnels and containers
Lettuces do well in poly-tunnels and containers, and are a good plant to have in a container by the back door. When it's time to plant out your young lettuces from the greenhouse or seed trays, plant a few in a container near the house, and early on in the year you can steal a leaf or two every day to pop into a sandwich or a small salad. Plant a few in a greenhouse or poly-tunnel and you'll have a few early salads.

Storing
Lettuces will store for 1 or 2 weeks in the refrigerator, but as it is high in water content, it's not advisable to try and store for any longer.

 Kale

History
Kale was the most common green vegetable in Europe up until the end of the Middle Ages and was cultivated by the ancient Romans as early as 600 BC. It was brought to America in the 17th century by the early settlers. The kale plant is a primitive form of cabbage but doesn't produce a 'head'. The leafy green plant has been cultivated in the home garden for at least 2000 years and is one of the most hardy of all winter vegetables.

Kale rarely suffers from diseases and pests. It tastes sweeter after the first frost, as do parsnips and brussels sprouts. For this reason, they are not as popular to grow in a warm climate. If your winters get cold though, kale is a great stand by vegetable and will last until early spring when other vegetables will be starting.

Growing Kale

Choosing kale ~ There are a number of different varieties of kale. The curly leaved variety is probably the most widely known, although seed is available for purple and flat-leaved kale as well. Some will be hardier than others and you should check seed packets carefully for growing instructions in your region to be sure of a good harvest. If you have the space, grow a couple of different types to help vary your winter diet.

When you buy your seed make sure you are buying edible kale, as there are ornamental varieties on the market that produce beautiful flowers and wonderful rockery-type plants, but are not good for eating.

Prepare the site ~ Kale likes to grow in a high nitrogen soil so it is advisable to use the same ground you used for early peas. The kale seed should be sown in early summer so there will be plenty of time to harvest the early peas. Don't dig the ground over. Just remove the weeds and hoe the lines where you will be sowing the seed.

The soil should retain a certain amount of moisture but also be well-drained. Brassicas tend to suffer from root diseases if the ground is too wet. As with other plants in this family, kale prefers to grow in soil that isn't too acidic, so if necessary, dig in a little lime to reduce the acid. However, kale is a much hardier brassica than most and is not as particular as cauliflower or cabbage. It will grow in much poorer soil.

Position ~ A bright, open site is fine but try to avoid windy places – the plants stay in the ground over winter and although they are frost resistant, a strong wind can damage most plants.

Sowing kale ~ Sow seed thinly in early summer. To produce a few autumn leaves for the stew pot, plant a line or two slightly earlier in the year. Thin out when the plants are about 3 in. (7 or 8 cm.) high, allowing a couple of inches (about 3 cm.) to grow.

When plants are about 6 in. (15 cm.) high, they are ready to transplant. Allow at least 12 in. (30 cm.) between plants. Double check your seed packets for exact spacing as some varieties will need more space than others. Water the plants the night before and transplant first thing in the morning for best results. Dig holes around 12 in. (30 cm.) apart and place 1 plant in each hole. Gently firm the soil around them. They should be planted so that the bottom leaves are just above the soil. Leave about 18 in. (45 cm.) between rows

If you live in a coastal area or the plants are in a particularly windy site, it may be a good idea to put in stakes to support the plants later on in the year. Push stake firmly in the ground to one side of the hole you have dug for your plant. Stakes shouldn't be put in after the plant is in the ground as they will damage the roots.

As soon as the plants have produced a few main leaves, a leaf or two can be picked from each plant, although kale does get sweeter after the first frost, so unless you really can't wait to try it, it is advisable to be patient. Kale can be harvested right up until the plant starts producing flowers, then it should be pulled up and composted. Depending on the type you grow, and the climate, kale can often have a new spurt of growth in early spring.

The plants can look a bit poorly during the winter, especially if they have had a few leaves taken here and there for the stew pot, but they tend to pick up well, and will normally carry on producing nourishing food for the family right through the winter months.

Caring for kale ~ One of the best things about winter vegetables is the lack of pests and diseases. Warm weather during the summer months breeds any number of viruses and bugs, but luckily in the winter that doesn't happen so much. Young kale plants could be at risk as they have to be planted in early summer so watch out for slugs and aphids. Later on in the summer, cabbage white butterflies could be a problem, but as the plants get established and the season wears on, there isn't too much else to worry about. Keep the plants weed-free as much as possible and well watered during long, dry spells.

In late summer or early autumn, if you haven't staked them, earth up your plants a little to protect them from wind or place a windbreak close by if the weather looks ominous. If you put in stakes when they were planted, use a natural fibre string and tie them gently to the stakes.

Poly-tunnels and containers
Kale shouldn't be protected against the frost as the taste improves in the cold weather. Growing under plastic will produce bitter plants.

Kale can be grown in containers but make sure they don't dry out. A couple of large containers next to the kitchen door can save trudging to the vegetable garden on wet winter days.

Storing
There isn't really any need to store kale as it grows through the winter and is readily available fresh when you need it. However, you can make a kale soup or stew and freeze in suitable containers. Remember to label with contents and date.

Pumpkin

History
Pumpkins date back many centuries and are native to Central America. They were originally known as a 'pepon', a Greek word meaning 'large melon'. The first pumpkin pies were created by carving out the seeds, filling the pumpkin case with honey, milk and spices, then baking in the ashes of a fire. They were also dried in strips, woven into rugs, and baked in long strips to be eaten by natives of Central America. Pumpkin seeds were eaten as part of a daily diet by many cultures. Pumpkin is a fruit and is generally harvested through the month of October. America is the largest producer.

Growing Pumpkin

Choosing your pumpkin ~ When buying your seed or plants, choose a sweet pumpkin and take the climate into consideration. Pumpkins need a fairly long growing season to fully develop and it's unlikely you'll be able to produce the huge varieties in a moderate climate unless you try growing them under glass. The smaller varieties are just as good to eat but you may have to buy your Halloween pumpkin if you're looking for a large one. Check on seed packets in your area and consider asking other pumpkin growers which varieties they value.

Prepare the site ~ I've only grown pumpkins on a flat patch, but many growers will say it's best to plant them on a hill that you create within your garden. Creating a mound will ensure good drainage, which is a good idea if you have heavy soil. Dig over the area and remove any stubborn weeds in the spring when weeds have just started to show themselves. Pumpkin plants need warm soil and lots of well-rotted manure dug into the ground in early spring, or the autumn before, to ensure the presence of good nutrients they thrive on.

Position ~ Pumpkins really do like hot, sunny spots and will tolerate a little shade during the hottest part of the day. The plants grow huge leaves, which help to shade the fruits. You will need to allow a lot of space for each plant as they tend to spread out. Follow the guidelines on the seed packet.

Sowing pumpkin ~ Pumpkin seeds need a fairly high temperature to germinate, and in many climates this means starting them off under glass or indoors. Some growers soak the seed in water for a few hours before sowing to encourage faster germination, but they will germinate without soaking. Check the growing advice on your seed packet, as every variety differs.

Start seeds in a fairly rich seed compost in small pots in the greenhouse or conservatory. They must have lots of light and warmth to get going. Keep the soil moist and watered every day but don't allow pots to become water-logged.

Once the ground is prepared, and there is no more chance of frost, the plants can be put outside. However, they must be big enough to withstand the move. The pumpkin plants should have at least two true leaves (not the first two), and the roots should be struggling to get out of the pots. Water each plant well and gently ease the plant out of its pot. With as little handling as possible, place in a prepared hole in your pumpkin patch. Firm down gently and water.

Leave a lot of space between plants – up to a metre is normal – to give them plenty of room to grow. When the baby plants first go outside, they tend to look rather forlorn and lonely, but don't be tempted to plant them closer together. They will grow towards each other soon enough. If it's still a little cold at night, consider covering the plants with a cloche to keep them as warm as possible in their early stages of development.

Caring for your pumpkin ~ Encourage frogs and toads to your garden as they keep slugs under control, and slugs adore young pumpkin plants.

When the fruits start to grow, place a board underneath each one to prevent them rotting from the earth, bugs and diseases.

Keep watered but never water-logged. In the early stages, keep a lookout for weeds. As the plants get bigger, weeds get little chance to grow under the enormous canopy of pumpkin leaves. I find so many frogs making their home under this canopy, it's almost impossible not to disturb them, and invariably while I check on the fruits, frogs are leaping out in indignant surprise!

Leave the pumpkins on the vine as long as possible and cut through the stem with a sharp knife when ready to harvest. The skin should be a good colour and hardened off. Cut when you are sure they have stopped growing.

Poly-tunnels and containers

Personally, I've never tried growing pumpkins indoors. I can't imagine finding the space! However, there is no reason why pumpkins shouldn't be grown in poly-tunnels or large cloches or even a greenhouse. If you are attempting to grow the super-large varieties, growing under glass or plastic would be preferable, especially in a moderate climate. Check with other growers in your region to see what they do.

Storing

Pumpkins will store for several months in the right conditions. While growing, your pumpkins need sun and water. In storage they need a dry, dark atmosphere. Bring pumpkins in the house when a frost is expected as they are **not** frost-hardy. Storing in a dry shed or garage is fine – but be wary of rodents. Mice love squashes, and one of your prize pumpkins will keep a whole family of mice happy for months. The best way to deter mice is to hang the pumpkins in nets from roof rafters or ceiling beams, being sure they don't touch each other. Many gardeners store vegetables like this.

Chapter Five

Growing Plants Rich in Vitamin B1

Broad beans, Garlic, Hazelnuts, Sweet corn

Broad Beans

History

Broad beans are one of the oldest foods cultivated in the western world. There is evidence that the broad bean was eaten around 6000BC in Israel but the bean didn't travel to the rest of Europe until around 3000BC.

Beans have always held many myths and legends and were believed at one time to be the souls of men who had previously died. High in protein, they were often eaten to replace meat. They were nearly always eaten with a grain to balance the lack of amino acids available in many types of bean.

In the middle ages, the French celebrated the twelfth day of Christmas with a cake called 'La Galette des Rois' (the Cake of Kings). A 'feve' (broad bean, which is a symbol of fertility) was baked inside the filling. The person who got the slice with the 'feve' was said to be blessed. Nowadays the custom is still enjoyed every year and the lucky person is crowned 'King for the Day'!

Growing Broad Beans

Choosing broad beans ~ Choose the broad bean variety to suit your region. Check with local growers if you are unsure which variety to use.

Some broad beans can be planted in autumn whilst others must be sown in spring. Reading the growing instructions on your seed packet is advisable as some hybrid varieties may be more suitable for spring or autumn sowing. If your soil is fairly heavy, spring sowings may be better; only plant in the autumn if your ground is very well-drained.

Prepare the site ~ Broad beans are fairly hardy and will grow in most soil types. If your soil is very acidic it's best to add a little lime before sowing. Deeply dug and prepared soil will yield a better crop. If possible, dig in some well-rotted manure or compost a few weeks before sowing, or in the previous autumn for spring sowings.

Many varieties of bean grow fairly tall and stakes can help the plants stay strong in the ground, especially for autumn sown plants. Windy spots are better avoided but stakes will help in any case. Position the stakes at regular intervals and tie a horizontal cane between them to create a more solid structure. Push the stakes firmly into the ground after digging and before sowing.

Position ~ Broad beans will grow best in full sun. However, beans are fairly hardy plants and have been known to grow and crop heavily next to hedges and in shady parts of the garden. Try a few in different places to see what works best.

Sowing broad beans ~ Broad beans are normally planted directly into the ground outside but if you want to get an early start on your spring crop, they can be started off in small pots, hardened off and then put out when the weather has improved. Use bio-degradable pots if possible. These pots are planted in the ground with the plant intact, which saves disturbing the roots. The pot naturally rots down and fertilises the soil.

The bean plant tends to be stronger when started off this way and is also likely to produce earlier beans. If the space is available, start a few plants in the greenhouse earlier in the year in biodegradable pots. Allow each plant a fair amount of space to develop; bean plants will grow happily in crowded conditions, but they will not crop as well.

Broad beans can be sown at intervals right through until June in most regions. Sow a line every couple of weeks or so to ensure a regular supply of fresh beans from spring through autumn.

Whole pods can be eaten when very young but other beans can be grown for this purpose. It seems a shame to eat the broad bean before it has fully developed as they are quite unique once mature: in taste, texture, nutrition and versatility.

Caring for broad beans ~ Black flies love broad beans and you should watch for the first signs of this fly getting hold of your bean crop. As soon as the plant is in full flower, taking the top 12–15 cm. off the plant will help prevent an attack of black fly. The tender, young leaves you take from the top of the plant can be eaten like spinach.

The plants need to be watered regularly and shouldn't be allowed to dry out. Keep a careful eye on your bean plants if the summer is particularly hot and dry.

Harvest a few young beans for your first taste of the year and let the main crop grow until there are five or more full size broad beans in each pod. If you have a good harvest it's worth leaving a few pods on the plant to completely mature and dry out. The beans inside can be stored and eaten during the winter months or you could save a few for sowing next year. Sowing beans you have grown yourself can result in a higher risk of disease in the plant, and care should be taken if you try this. However, it often works perfectly and will also benefit your pocket.

When the beans have been harvested, cut the plant down to ground level and compost. Burn if there are any signs of disease. Dig the roots of healthy plants back into the ground, but pull up the roots of the unhealthy ones. Peas and beans have properties that help fix nitrogen into the soil and digging the nitrogen fixing roots back into the soil will benefit the crop you grow on this ground the following season.

Beans shouldn't be grown on the same spot every year. It's always a good idea to rotate your crops, and the pea and bean patch is better grown on fresh soil for 3–4 years before returning to the original patch. This goes for most annual vegetables, while perennial crops such as asparagus remain in the same place for many years.

Poly-tunnels and containers
Broad beans are happy to grow in full sun and are self-pollinating so they should be okay to grow inside. It is worth growing autumn sowing varieties indoors if your region suffers heavy frosts or extreme cold during the winter months, but watch out for humidity and aphids. Hoe regularly around the plants, as the soil in poly-tunnels can get stale and develop fungus, which in turn can affect your bean plants.

Storing
Beans are probably one of the best vegetables to store as they will keep indefinitely once dried. Leave on the plant until the pod is starting to shrivel and is about to open and shed the beans. (If the weather is particularly wet, harvest the beans and dry on a rack in a very slow oven for a couple of hours.) Collect and store in a dry place, preferably in a glass jar. Keep away from direct sunlight and moisture.

Fresh beans can be frozen successfully and kept for a long period of time. Shell the beans, lay them on trays and freeze quickly. Put into sealable containers or bags and label before storing in the freezer. Broad beans can also be canned or bottled if you have the equipment at home for processing.

 Garlic

History
Garlic has been cultivated and used as a food flavouring and healing herb for at least 5000 years; there is evidence of use by the ancient Egyptians. Garlic is said to have originated in Asia and has been used as a food additive and to treat various ailments around the globe. It was thought, at one time, to be a powerful aphrodisiac, and therefore not considered suitable for monks, young women or anyone who should not be arousing their passions! Garlic wasn't considered to be a socially acceptable food for the upper classes because of its strong odour. For many centuries, Buddhists believed that garlic should not be taken as a food, but simply used as a healing herb; however, garlic and other strong tasting herbs are now used in cooking throughout India.

Garlic is believed to have strong cleansing properties and is a healthy addition to the modern diet. However, it can aggravate certain conditions, such as eczema, and should be eaten in moderation by those suffering from such conditions. Garlic is a useful healing herb and syrup of garlic, made by pouring boiling water over fresh sliced cloves and leaving overnight, helps cure coughs, asthma, bronchitis and other chest or lung illnesses.

There are many myths and legends attached to garlic. It has been believed that garlic hung by the front door will ward off sickness as well as vampires!

Growing garlic

·Choosing garlic ~ Buy garlic from your garden centre or local nursery. Although, in the garden, nothing can be guaranteed, I have found planting any old garlic works fine. You can plant any time from mid December to late February, depending on the weather. Garlic will tolerate the cold.

Prepare the site ~ Because garlic can be planted very early in the year, it's a good idea to prepare the ground at the end of the autumn just before the cold or very wet weather sets in. Dig over, remove all the weeds and add in some well-rotted organic manure or compost. Cover the ground with black plastic or similar covering until you are ready to plant the garlic cloves. Garlic prefers a sandy, moist soil but will grow in most soils. Dig in a little lime if you have a very acid soil.

Position ~ Although garlic will tolerate the cold, it is predominantly a warm weather plant and will benefit from a sunny position. When preparing the ground in the autumn, make sure it's a sunny spot to get the best harvest possible.

Planting garlic ~ Garlic has been traditionally planted on the shortest day of the year; in the northern hemisphere that would be just before Christmas on winter solstice. February or March are also reasonable months to plant garlic, and with a good summer, they could still be ready to harvest in August or September.

Separate the cloves and plant the healthiest in firm ground about 2 in. (5 cm.) deep. Try not to leave the top of the cloves poking out of the ground as the birds may steal them. Leave about 6 in. (15 cm.) between cloves and about 12 in. (30 cm.) between rows. Plant as many as your space allows. Garlic stores well so you can always use a good harvest.

Caring for garlic ~ Water and keep weeded especially during the early spring while the cloves are getting established and putting down their roots. During the summer months, garlic needs watering and keeping as weed free as possible, but generally it will just get on with growing all by itself. Pests don't seem to like it very much. Maybe the strong odour puts them off!

Sometimes the plants put up a solid stalk that produces a flower. This won't affect the taste or condition of the bulb apart from perhaps a clove or two being too 'woody'. Some gardeners prefer to snap these stalks off or fold them down like onions, but I just leave them.

When the leaves start to wither and dry, they are almost ready to pull up. Leave for a day or two until the leaves have almost lost all green colour. Fork around each bulb carefully to avoid damage and lift on a sunny day. Lay the garlic on the dry earth for a couple of hours, turning now and then to dry them evenly.

Poly-tunnels and containers

I've tried to grow garlic in containers a few times but never had any success. I can only presume they like to be in the open or alongside fellow cloves.

Garlic can be grown in a poly-tunnel but make sure there is a good air supply and that you hoe around the cloves from time to time so that the bulb can mature without weeds or any moulds getting in the way. Because the environment in a poly-tunnel can be humid, the soil can become stale and various fungi can develop. Make sure the ground is well watered and there is a good air supply and you should be able to produce a good crop of garlic.

Storing

Garlic will store well right through the winter months if dried properly. Dry in the sun for a few hours after digging up. Then hang for a few days to a week until the earth can be easily brushed off. Don't wash the garlic bulbs. They need to be kept dry if you want to store them for any length of time. Once they have dried and the earth has been removed, string or plait them in lengths of 12–20 bulbs. Try not to let the bulbs press against each other as they will deteriorate more quickly.

Hang plaits or strings of garlic in a dark, dry place for the winter. Keep one plait in the corner of the kitchen. It is convenient and gives the kitchen an air of French cuisine, always encouraging for the chef.

Hazelnuts

History

Nuts have always been eaten by man. Fruit and nuts were gathered and formed the major part of our diet when meat or fish was unavailable. Nuts are seeds with a hard shell and so store well during winter months. Many animals store nuts for the winter hibernation period. The squirrel is probably the best known animal to store nuts. And anyone who has ever tried growing hazelnuts in their garden will know they have to be very quick to harvest the nuts before the squirrels arrive. Nuts have been cultivated for many centuries. Most nuts are the seed of trees and will develop into new trees when the nut is planted.

Growing Hazelnuts

Choosing hazelnuts ~ Many different nuts can be grown in a domestic garden, depending on the space you have available and the climate. Local growers are a good starting place for information. Your local nursery is likely to be selling the trees that will grow successfully in your area. Visit them to ask what varieties they suggest.

Once you are aware of the trees that will grow well in your part of the world, it's really a case of deciding whether you have space for them. There are many hybrid plants available now in dwarf form, and you will probably be able to buy a number of trees that will stay fairly small but will still provide a good crop of nuts every year.

If you don't like the hybrid idea, it's still possible to grow workable trees in an orchard space. Keep them trimmed every year and look after them well so you can collect the nuts rather than having to leave them to the squirrels. Hazel grows well as a hedgerow crop.

Prepare the site ~ Because of their size and special needs, preparing your site for nut trees can be very complicated. I believe the rule of thumb should be 'simple but effective'. If you have done adequate preparation, it's likely that the trees you have chosen will be happy in your garden and will produce a very nice harvest.

When you buy your individual trees, make sure you have full planting instructions from the nursery so you know whether your tree requires acid or well-drained soil, how much space to allow, and whether they prefer full sun, part shade or a sheltered position.

Position ~ It's a good idea to do a little research and find out how your trees will develop. Generally, it's not a good idea to plant trees too close to your house or other buildings as tree roots can play havoc with foundations and drains. If the tree grows very large, it can block the sun from your house.

Unless you are growing trees that produce pine nuts (which are generally too large to grow near the house anyway), deciduous nut trees will shed their leaves in autumn. This colourful mess can be pretty for a few days, but as soon as the rain or snow arrives, you'll be raking slushy, slippery leaves every day. Keeping a patch of land especially for your orchard trees, whether fruit or nuts, keeps the mess to one place and you won't need to rake all the time.

Planting hazelnuts ~ All trees take a number of years to develop enough to produce a fruit or seed. Some will take ten years or more and most of us don't want to wait that long to start harvesting our first crop of nuts. Many trees you buy in a garden centre or local tree supplier will be grafted — the tree has been combined with an older, hardier tree that will support its growth and help it develop to maturity sooner. These are a very good way of starting your nut orchard and should not be ignored.

Follow the planting instructions that come with your tree. Generally, a large enough hole should be dug in a bright, sunny spot and well-rotted manure dug deep into the soil. Tease the roots of your tree apart gently and place into the hole. Fill with the soil you dug out and firm down with your heel. Water well and keep watered especially during the first growing season. Keep any strong perennial weeds out of the way and make sure the ground doesn't get water-logged.

Cuttings also work for some trees. I have grown many new hazel trees from cuttings simply pushed into the ground in the autumn and left to their own devices. You may wish to dip the rooting end in a hormone powder before planting. Many growers swear by this method as the only sure way of getting your cuttings to produce the roots they need quickly enough for next year's growing season. Experimenting with cuttings can be fun and inexpensive, but the success rate may be lower than other methods of growing new trees.

Planting trees is always a good thing to do, and you could try growing hazel along with willow to form hedgerows. Mixed hedgerows are very attractive to the eye and to wildlife. Birds will nest more readily in a mixed hedgerow than a regular leylandii or privet hedge. Encouraging birds to your garden is fine as long as you aren't growing soft fruits or green, leafy vegetables.

Caring for hazelnuts ~ Caring for trees generally takes less maintenance time than caring for a vegetable patch. However, until well established, trees should be kept as healthy as possible. This short checklist should be all you need to produce a crop of nuts every year:

- keep surrounding areas free of perennial weeds
- ensure ground is not water-logged at any time of the year
- water well during long, dry periods
- keep an eye on the general health of your tree; regularly check for any bugs and viruses and treat if necessary
- prune once or twice a year according to growing instructions for your particular tree
- harvest nuts before the squirrels get them!

Poly-tunnels and containers

Trees aren't really very suitable for indoor growing. They can be grown in poly-tunnels and large greenhouses if kept small and manageable. But generally trees thrive outdoors and they provide homes for many birds and insects.

Storing

Nuts are probably one of the best foods we can store and certainly the easiest. Their hard shell keeps them from harm and they will keep for many months during the winter if kept dry and out of direct sunlight. Look over all the nuts before storing. Check for:

- small holes in the shell – they could be housing a bug or two
- any sign of mould – mould spreads quickly
- distorted shapes – could be due to a virus

Remove any less-than-perfect specimens and discard. Store the rest in net bags or spread out in plastic or wooden trays. Don't keep too many in one place just in case you missed a problem or dampness causes mould to set in. Keep the nuts as dry as you can and in a fairly dark place. A cupboard is okay but it shouldn't be too warm as the nut inside the shell will dry out and become inedible. Keep away from mice, squirrels and any other vermin or nut thieves.

Sweet corn

History

Corn or maize has its roots in prehistoric times but not the sweet corn variety that we enjoy today; that was bred more recently from other corn varieties. Maize has been one of the main staples of the human diet for thousands of years and is a cereal. It is the third most grown cereal crop after wheat and rice.

Thought to have originated in South America, corn quickly spread all over the globe and is a useful food crop today, especially for those who have intolerance to wheat products; corn makes an excellent alternative. There is documented evidence of sweet corn as early as 1800 and was probably grown by the native South Americans. Sweet corn wasn't cultivated on a commercial level until the 1950s and since then the development of hybrid varieties enable all gardeners to successfully grow their own crop.

Growing sweet corn

Choosing sweet corn ~ Buy the variety that grows well in your area. Your local garden centre or nursery will be able to advise you or ask local gardeners for their tips and advice. Some hybrid varieties are more suitable to shorter growing seasons and some are shorter in height and will grow successfully in a windy spot. New seed should be used every year. If you decide to grow different varieties you could have a cross-pollination problem. To get around this, different types of corn should have at least 250 feet or approximately 80 metres of space between them.

Prepare the site ~ Sweet corn isn't too fussy about the soil but it won't grow well in heavy clay or very wet soil. The roots go deep so the area should be deeply turned before planting, and if you can, dig in some well-rotted compost or manure to give it an extra boost during the growing season. Remove all perennial weeds and any non-organic debris from the soil.

Position ~ Sweet corn is pollinated by the wind although it doesn't like an exposed and windy position. Make sure the area is well sheltered to avoid wind damage. Find a spot in full sun and allow at least a four foot or one and a half metre block for growing 12–15 plants.

Sowing sweet corn ~ Sweet corn plants don't like to be transplanted but in a moderate climate you will need to start the seeds early in the year, as they need a fairly long growing season to fully develop the corncobs. Therefore in a cooler climate plant your seeds in bio-degradable pots that can be planted in the ground later without disturbing the roots.

Start the seeds in early spring, sowing 1–3 seeds per pot (check on your seed packet for full instructions). When the seedlings start to grow, carefully remove the weaker plants leaving one plant per pot to continue. Keep warm and watered until all threat of frost has passed and the ground outside has warmed up.

Transplant your corn outside in blocks to allow for pollination, as sweet corn grown in long rows won't produce cobs. Allow around 40–50 cm. growing space for each plant. If you sow the seed directly outside, plant every 20–30 cm. and remove weaker plants if necessary.

In a temperate to warm climate, sweet corn can be planted twice or even three times during the year, giving a regular supply of corn for many months. It may also be planted directly outside instead of starting the seed in a greenhouse.

In a moderate climate corn needs a longer growing season and it's unlikely you'll be able to produce more than one harvest of sweet corn per year.

Caring for sweet corn ~ Keep sweet corn clear of weeds and water thoroughly. The soil must be well-drained or the roots will rot very quickly. Watch for wind damage. Ideally your corn will be positioned out of any strong wind currents. Keep an eye on your plants for any diseases or pests and treat as soon as you can.

Corncobs should be harvested during the 'milky' stage. Gently peel back the leaf around the cob and lightly press on a kernel. If a milky substance is released, the corn is ready to eat. This stage only lasts around three weeks and the cobs should be checked regularly to avoid leaving them too long on the plant. The silky tassels start turning brown when the corn is ripening.

The cob should be snapped downwards and twisted slightly to remove from the main plant and eaten as soon as possible. Hold the main stem of the plant firmly to avoid damage if there are other cobs to collect later. When all cobs have been collected, pull plants and break into smaller lengths before composting or burning.

Poly-tunnels and containers

As sweet corn needs to be pollinated by the wind, indoor growing would prove difficult. However, nothing's impossible. Check with your seed supplier for new hybrid varieties and look into local growing techniques for indoor growing.

Storing

Sweet corn really is best eaten very fresh. The natural sugars turn to starch fairly quickly and a cob bought from the supermarket will be less nutritious than the cob picked from your garden and eaten on the same day. There will be a noticeable difference in taste too.

However, if you leave the outer leaves round the cob it can be stored successfully in the fridge for a few days. And if the processing is carried out very quickly after picking, sweet corn can be frozen, canned or bottled and maintain nearly all its vitamin content and taste. To freeze corn, strip the kernels from the cob, place on trays and freeze quickly. Put into bags or containers and label.

Chapter Six

Growing Plants Rich in Vitamin B2

Mushrooms, Salsify, Spinach, Watercress

Mushrooms

History

Mushrooms have been a plant of wonder for thousands of years. There is evidence that fungi were eaten during the stone age and the ancient Egyptians believed they were fit only for royalty; common people were not allowed to touch them. All sorts of myths have been attached to mushrooms – from immortality to umbrellas for leprechauns! In some parts of the world, mushrooms had a bad reputation for many years, probably due to some varieties being hallucinogenic or deadly.

It wasn't until the 17th century that fungi became more commonly cultivated, but it took the entrepreneurs of the early 19th century to get the mushroom industry up and running. In the early days mushrooms were grown under other plants and were a secondary crop, making them unavailable for a large part of the year. Modern day techniques ensure we can put mushrooms on our table every day. We can even buy ready-to-grow kits to grow mushrooms in our own homes.

Growing mushrooms

Choosing mushrooms ~ Growing mushrooms in kit form is somewhat limiting but a good start on the ladder to being a fungi expert. The white mushrooms we buy in packs in the supermarket are the most common type to grow yourself, and they often produce a lot more than you expect. Otherwise spores can be bought from specialist suppliers ready to inject into your growing medium.

Prepare the site ~ Fungi lives under leaves, in grassland, under the bark of trees and anywhere else that suits it.

When conditions are right, the fungi will produce a mushroom, which starts to deteriorate almost as soon as it's fully grown and therefore should be picked and eaten while still young.

Wine growers have to be very precise in the timing of their grape harvest and the mushroom grower needs to develop that same skill. Luckily it's not that hard. It is fascinating to watch how they develop and decay. It all happens over the course of a couple of days. Cultivating mushrooms from a kit will demonstrate the life cycle beautifully. The three stages are:

- spawning: the spawn is established in a growing medium
- pinning: tiny pin heads of mycelium appear
- fruiting: the developing mushroom

Position ~ Some mushrooms may need a little light at times, others will grow in very shady spots. A little patch of woodland in your garden area will really help with outside growing. Otherwise, spawn can be injected into an old tree trunk and can be an interesting feature of your garden. You may need to experiment a little before you get the conditions absolutely right for your mushrooms.

Sowing mushrooms ~ Although mushrooms are classified as fungi, they need the right growing conditions, as all plants do, to produce a bumper crop. Mushrooms are just as nutritious as vegetables and don't have to be treated as a luxury crop. They have their own particular seasons, and different species of fungi require different conditions to thrive.

Collecting wild mushrooms

There are hundreds of different species of fungi. Fungi have an important role to play in the natural world around us. Some aid growth of other plants and trees and some will poison those same plants. **Never eat any form of fungi without a positive identification first. Some wild fungi are highly poisonous and can cause convulsions and death.**

Once you know what to look for, collecting wild mushrooms for food is a rewarding and tasty experience. As a family, we have collected and eaten chanterelles, giant puff balls, shaggy ink caps, field mushrooms, and, my particular favourite, chicken-of-the-woods. The chicken-of-the-woods fungi live on the bark of trees like the beefsteak fungi. One sizeable chicken-of-the-woods will feed a family for 2 days. And it really is delicious!

Caring for mushrooms ~ If you've never grown mushrooms, a kit really will help with the fungi-growing learning curve. Each stage of development requires different conditions. Button varieties will develop without light, while other species may require light during one or more of its stages of development.

Mushrooms can also be grown in those out of the way, dark corners in the garden, where nothing else will grow. Many varieties can be grown outside in mild climates. They rarely cope with very low temperatures and should be grown indoors during cold weather conditions.

Poly-tunnels and containers

Try an indoor growing kit. Poly-tunnels tend to be warm and humid and an ideal growing space for all kinds of fungi.

Storing
Mushrooms can be frozen, bottled or dried. Bottling requires the right equipment but if you are set up for this process, mushrooms can be stored for many months without losing any of their flavour. Textures tend to change with bottled mushrooms but this happens with any stored product compared with the fresh original.

Freezing ~ Quick-freeze whole or sliced mushrooms on a tray, then store in bags or plastic containers. Label and put in the freezer immediately. Frozen mushrooms will keep for many months.

Drying ~ Drying mushrooms is the most popular form of storing. Many chefs will prefer to use dried rather than fresh mushrooms as the flavour tends to be more intense. Slice mushrooms or keep them whole if fairly thin, and thread onto a length of cotton thread with a regular sewing needle. Hang this over a stove or in an airing cupboard for about eight hours or until very dry. Label and store in a glass jar or sealable bag.

Mushrooms can be dried in a food dryer or in a simple home-made drying area. Rig up a light bulb in the bottom of a cardboard box and attach trays above it. Spread mushrooms on the trays and plug in the light for a few hours. A very simple idea but it works! Make sure mushrooms are entirely dry before storing.

Salsify

History
The ancient Romans and Greeks used to collect wild salsify over 2000 years ago; the stems and roots of some varieties were eaten. The stems resemble asparagus. Salsify and it's close relative scorzonera (black salsify) weren't cultivated until the middle ages and since then have gone in and out of fashion in the home vegetable garden. It produces an attractive flower and can be grown in borders and still be used as a good standby vegetable in the early winter months. Salsify will stay in the ground for most of the winter months and depending on your climate, could still be edible in the early spring.

Salsify has been called 'the oyster plant' because of its oyster-like taste. Scorzonera is black skinned and has a stronger flavour.

Growing salsify
Choosing salsify ~ Choose a hardy variety for your region. Salsify is an annual plant and will flower, seed and then die. Scorzonera is a perennial and will keep growing through the second year and produce wider and longer roots.

Prepare the site ~ Salsify prefers a neutral soil rather than acid or alkaline. The soil should be deeply worked for the roots to develop properly. Fresh manure causes roots to fork and shouldn't be added to the ground where any root crops will be grown. Remove large stones and rocks from the ground, as well as any perennial weeds and non-organic debris.

Position ~ Salsify is a very hardy plant and will probably grow almost anywhere in your garden, as long as the soil is well-drained. Try growing a line in full sun and another in part shade and compare the two. Certain hybrid varieties will be more adapted to climatic conditions in your region than others.

Sowing salsify ~ Salsify seed can be planted as soon as the ground becomes workable after the winter months. A few frosts early in their growing cycle will improve the taste and harvest.

After the ground has been deeply dug and cleaned of weeds and stones, gently hoe a line for your seed. Make a shallow trench about 1 in. (2.5 cm.) deep and plant the salsify seed. Cover with fine soil and water gently.

Leave about 12 in. (30 cm.) between rows. Salsify can easily be mistaken for grass. Make sure you know where your seeds are sown and don't pull out the new salsify plants thinking they are small clumps of grass.

Thin out after a few weeks when the plants seem like they're starting to overcrowd.

Allow 8–12 in. (20–30 cm.) for each plant to grow. The plants you remove should be added to the compost. Root crops don't tend to transplant very well, and if they do get going, the roots tend to be forked and not as easy to prepare in the kitchen.

Salsify seed is very unlikely to last more than one year so plant all your seed and buy fresh each year. You may be able to collect some seed from your own plants later in the year. Wait for the flowers and observe when they produce seed. Some hybrids won't produce any seed or it will be inferior quality, but it is always worth trying to get your own seed if you can. Salsify will die after producing flowers and seeds so just leave a few plants for seed collecting and eat the rest.

Caring for salsify ~ Salsify is a hardy plant and shouldn't need much looking after. Water regularly and keep weed-free but apart from that your salsify plants should just get on with it themselves. They don't tend to suffer with any pests either. They can be left in the ground during the winter and dug up for eating in the spring. Dig very deeply and carefully with a fork when lifting salsify to avoid damage to the roots.

Poly-tunnels and containers

Salsify isn't suitable for indoor growing. It is a hardy plant and will stand up to most climatic conditions. There isn't really much point in using up precious poly-tunnel or greenhouse space to grow this crop.

The roots go very deep and if you use containers, they will have to be very deep as well. Salsify can be as long as 12 in. (30 cm.) and the container will have to be about twice that depth to allow for root growth and full development.

Storing

In late autumn before the ground freezes – if it does in your part of the world – dig up as much salsify as you want to eat before the thaw. Twist off the tops and store in a dry, dark place. Salsify should be treated like carrots and either hung in sacks, making sure they are dry first, or in mouse-proof barrels of sand. Later, when the ground thaws, the other roots can be dug up and eaten. In mild winter regions, the salsify roots can be left in the ground all winter and used as required.

Spinach

History

Spinach was used more than 2000 years ago in southwest Asia, in the region around Persia. In the 7th century, spinach was introduced to China and was imported to Spain in the 12th century. It wasn't until the 13th century that spinach became a useful vegetable to grow in Europe. It travelled slowly until it reached America in the early 19th century. It is still widely collected as a wild, green, leafy vegetable in the Mediterranean area. In 1920, Popeye the Sailor man was a cartoon character used to push spinach onto the unsuspecting American public and it worked very well!

Growing Spinach

Choosing spinach ~ Spinach belongs to the same family as chard, which is often grown in moderate or warm summer climates because it doesn't bolt or run to seed as quickly as spinach. Choose a variety that is compatible with your climate and check seed packets before you buy. Some traditional spinach varieties won't tolerate any hot, sunny days and will bolt within hours of the sun coming out. Growing in shady areas may help, but it's probably better to choose a variety more suitable to warm weather if that's where you live.

Prepare the site ~ In cooler climates, choose a fairly light place in your garden, otherwise position partly in shade. Dig in well-rotted manure, preferably at least one season before you intend to plant your spinach, and work the soil to around 12 in. deep. The spinach plant has a long taproot and will grow well if the soil has been cleaned fairly deeply. Make sure the soil is well-drained, and not too acidic; if you suspect your soil is high in acid content, add lime or other neutralising products to adjust the PH levels.

Position ~ It's best to go for a shadier spot if you live in a fairly warm climate. Rows of spinach plants will thrive in a healthy vegetable plot, but there's no reason why spinach or chard plants can't be grown individually in odd places around the garden.

Sowing spinach ~ Start your spinach seeds off directly outside up to 8 weeks before the last frost. Check on the seed packet for regional variations. Sowing in late winter/early spring will give you a crop of spinach early in the summer before the lettuces are ready to pick.

Seed should be sown about half an inch deep and kept watered and weeded while germination occurs. Germination takes around one to two weeks depending on the variety and weather conditions. Try to sow the seed thinly so you don't have to do too much thinning later.

Caring for spinach ~ Once the spinach plants are about 4 in. (10 cm.) tall, they will need to be thinned. Remove every other plant and toss the baby plants into a salad bowl. Young plants are highly nutritious and should be enjoyed after your hard work in the garden. 2–3 weeks later, you should thin them again.

The final plot should support one spinach plant every 15–30 cm. depending again on the variety. Read your seed packets for space allowances.

Be aware of pests! Slugs aren't as keen on spinach as they are on lettuce, BUT they will eat anything that's available, so be vigilant. Try spreading broken egg shells around your plants.

As well as slugs, birds can be a problem in the vegetable garden. I always had trouble with birds nibbling the leaves of my young spinach plants. A little is okay but keep an eye on them: unchecked, they will call all their friends and turn your plot into an 'all-you-can-eat' buffet for birds!

Old CDs or DVDs strung between posts make great deterrents for birds. Cats also work quite well, however they can also chase away beneficial frogs and toads and are very fond of sunning themselves on your newly dug and seeded rows in the vegetable garden!

Poly-tunnels and containers

Although spinach is not a particularly good plant for warm climates, the problem is usually because of direct sun sending them to seed too soon. Try out a few plants on the windowsill or in a bright room in your house, but avoid direct sunlight. Poly-tunnels could prove to be too bright but a greenhouse with whitewashed glass will produce a good spinach crop. Remember to keep it well watered. Containers are fine for spinach, as long as they are deep, well-drained and watered regularly.

Storing

Spinach leaves can be stored in a plastic bag in the fridge for a few days. Don't wash the leaves and store them as dry as possible. Spinach can also be frozen but the texture will change dramatically when thawed. Use when spinach is only partly thawed to save texture being too soft and slushy. Otherwise spinach is very much a fresh vegetable and is best eaten in season rather than kept for too long.

Watercress

History

Watercress has been cultivated for at least 2000 years. It was always considered to be a herb with special healing powers. Throughout history, soldiers have been given watercress as part of their diet to increase their strength; it was also believed to help growth in young children. Most leafy, green vegetables are high in mineral and vitamin content and watercress is no exception.

Watercress originates in Asia and the Mediterranean area and wasn't cultivated in Europe until the Middle Ages. In England the first commercial production of watercress didn't occur until early in the 19th century.

It has always been thought that watercress will only grow in running water but it will grow successfully in very moist soil. It's also an ideal plant to add to a water feature. The constant running water of a fountain or pond in a home garden is an ideal place to grow watercress. Practical and attractive, it will enhance the feature in your garden.

Watercress can become contaminated with 'liver fluke' – a fatal disease – from the droppings of cows and sheep. Water carries the disease quickly and if you live close to these animals you will need to take extra care. Never pick wild watercress if there is a farm nearby.

Growing Watercress

Choosing watercress ~ Seeds can be bought, but sometimes you'll find a bunch of watercress from the market that has a few straggly roots. These are good starting plants for your watercress crop. It's also possible to grow a few roots on a stem yourself. Place a stalk in a small jar of water for a week or two, changing the water regularly. If nothing happens, either eat or discard, but if you find a few fine roots, persevere until the roots look strong enough to be planted in soil.

Prepare the site ~ If you have a water feature in your garden with a slow running stream of water, that will probably be your best site for watercress. Otherwise, a number of other ways are possible. If you have an outside tap on the side of your house, you can create a convenient watercress site. Bury a length of guttering up to the rim and pour in a thin layer of gravel. Top that with a good potting or seed compost or fertile soil from the garden, and you have the perfect place for your watercress. Or create a watercress pond by sinking an old paddling pool into the vegetable garden, making sure there are holes in the bottom for drainage. Again put in a layer of gravel and water. Sink trays of watercress in the water.

Position ~ Full sun isn't necessary but watercress will thrive in a fairly sunny spot. It needs warmth but not too much humidity. A few experiments may be necessary to find the right spot in your garden, especially with the needs of watercress being slightly special. A well positioned bed under an outside tap, a paddling pool or water feature are all reasonable possibilities as long as they're not in deep shade or full sun all day.

Sowing watercress ~ See 'Choosing watercress' above for alternate ways to start watercress. Otherwise, start off your plants the regular way and plant some seed. Start the seeds off in a fairly rich organic seed compost or good soil from the garden. Watercress doesn't like acid soil. Sow the seeds in trays or small pots and keep moist at all times. Never let the soil dry out. When the plants have a few true leaves, and the weather is warm enough, they'll be ready to plant outside.

Another way to germinate the seeds is to lay a paper towel on a flat tray and sprinkle the seeds onto it. Keep the towel wet at all times and look after it indoors until the plants are ready to put out in the garden. The seeds should germinate within a couple of weeks. As soon as they germinate, they should be placed in pots of soil and after another 10 days to 2 weeks, the young seedlings will be ready to transplant. During all stages of development and growth, watercress must be kept wet. Plant out in the garden in your preferred site leaving each plant about 8 in. (20 cm.) of space all round.

Caring for watercress ~ Watercress is a hardy perennial and once established it doesn't really need any looking after, if it always has a fresh water supply. It's a wonderful cut-and-come-again plant. Cut stems back to just above ground level and the roots will push up fresh shoots. The best time to eat watercress is in slightly cooler weather as it tends to get limp and less tasty during hot summer days. Watercress flowers from May to September and the tiny flowers are very attractive either in the pond, next to your house or in the middle of the vegetable patch.

Poly-tunnels and containers
Warning, if you live near a farm with cows and sheep, care must be taken in growing watercress, therefore container growing is the best option. Creating a running water system in a poly-tunnel or greenhouse is ideal, although watercress is at its best during the cooler parts of the year so the temperature will need to be controlled. If you need to keep your greenhouse or tunnel very warm, outside growing would be advisable. Watercress will have to be grown in containers of some sort, whether it be very wet soil in pots, or a garden pond. It can become invasive given the right conditions, so keep eating it!

Storing
Watercress can be stored for a few days in the refrigerator but is really best eaten fresh. Or use watercress in a recipe and freeze the whole dish, such as watercress soup. Make the soup, cool thoroughly and pour into a suitable container. Label and freeze immediately.

Chapter Seven

Growing Plants Rich in Vitamin B6

Cabbage, Celeriac, Onions, Potatoes

History

Cabbage originated in the Mediterranean region and has been eaten for more than 3000 years. By around 200BC the cabbage was being cultivated as a food crop. The Chinese cabbage may have been cultivated for even longer than the European types. Over the centuries many different medicinal attributes have been linked to cabbage: from helping milk production in nursing mothers to hangover cures.

Cabbage was introduced to the Americas in the early 16th century and quickly became a popular vegetable. Because it grows fairly quickly, has many different varieties, and can be grown and/or stored for most of the year, the cabbage has become a staple in the diet of many countries, in particular, northern and colder climates. Pound for pound the cabbage produces more food per acre than practically any other cultivated vegetable.

Sauerkraut (cabbage preserved in brine) was an important food on many sea voyages and has kept generations of families healthy enough to survive harsh, northern winters in Russia and Germany.

Myths, legends and folklore have been attached to cabbages over many centuries, Children of past generations were even told that babies came from the cabbage patch!

Growing cabbage

Choosing cabbage ~ There are hundreds of different varieties of cabbage, with new and traditional types turning up every few years. They are available in all shapes, sizes and colours from almost white through different greens, purples and reds. They can be soft and leafy or have very solid heads that are round or conical in shape. Cabbage can be eaten raw but not all varieties taste particularly good that way. White cabbage is probably the best cabbage to eat raw and is the main ingredient in coleslaw.

Most cabbage varieties will bolt during very hot weather and if you live in a particularly warm climate, choose a variety that will mature before the hot weather arrives. Look on seed packets for growing conditions required for your region. Some types are happier in certain regions, and you'll find your local nursery or garden centre will stock regional favourites. Chat with cabbage growers locally and find out what they grow.

It's nice to grow a mixture of vegetables, and the same goes for a particular vegetable. If you have rows and rows of Savoy cabbages all maturing at once, however tasty they are, the family will undoubtedly get bored with them. Vary the types you grow. You may also experiment a little without the risk of losing a large crop through adverse weather or soil conditions.

Prepare the site ~ Cabbages are greedy feeders and it's best to dig in some well-rotted manure or compost earlier in the year so that when you plant out your small cabbage plants they will have a good start. As with many plants, cabbages need plenty of water, especially in the early weeks of growth. Find a spot that's well-drained but retains a certain amount of water so the soil feels fairly moist most of the time. The ground should be dug over and large stones and perennial weeds removed. Break up the soil to a fairly fine consistency, although it doesn't have to be as fine as if you were sowing carrots or tomatoes.

Position ~ Most varieties of cabbage don't need full sun, although you should check on the seed packets for specific variety needs. They will need light so best not to choose a very shady spot. I prefer to grow a few cabbages here and there in the garden, mostly to confuse the cabbage white butterfly. The 'cabbage white' will lay her eggs and the resulting caterpillars can destroy a whole cabbage patch in a couple of days, so if you can do anything to avoid this, try it!

Sowing cabbage ~ Buying small plants ready for planting out is the quickest and easiest way to get your cabbage patch up and running. Buy from a local supplier as these varieties will be more likely to be happy in your region.

Otherwise, starting from seed isn't difficult and is a lot more rewarding. Choose a few different varieties, such as a white cabbage, a Savoy and maybe a red or Chinese variety.

Prepare a seed tray in your greenhouse or other warm place and plant your seed in a fairly rich seed compost. Keep watered and look after them for a few weeks until the seedlings are around 5–10 cm. tall (check on your packets for individual growing instructions). If you are growing a few different types, remember to label each tray.

Don't let your cabbage plants dry out as this will seriously stunt their growth. A cabbage is 90% water and needs a constant water supply. (In a high rainfall area, as long as the ground is well-drained, cabbages tend to do very well.) When your seedlings are ready to plant out, dig a fairly large hole for each plant, allowing about 60 cm. between plants and between rows. Double check on your seed packets again, as the conical shapes need less space than the huge leafy types.

Place the plant into the hole and fill with a mixture of compost and the soil you dug out. Firm down gently and water well.

Caring for cabbage ~ Keep your cabbage plants well watered, especially during hot, dry weather. If cabbages are fed well, they will develop into a high source of nutrition. A natural feed made from comfrey and nettles works well. In a container with a lid, cover comfrey and nettle leaves with water for a few weeks, then drain off the liquid and pour onto your vegetable patch. The liquid acts as a tonic for the soil and helps the plants extract nutrients a lot easier. Hold your breath before opening because the smell will be horrendous. You can repeat this treatment every few weeks if you have the comfrey and nettles available. Comfrey is a respected green manure and won't hurt your plants at all, and you can use it without the nettles. Nettles are a good supplement though as they're also high in vitamins and iron. If you haven't the comfrey available buy an organic fertiliser for your cabbages and apply every couple of weeks, or according to the manufacturer's recommendation.

While your plants are young, watch out for wind damage. If they get blown about too much, the stem can break and the plant will die. Use a temporary windbreak if the wind is exceptionally harsh. A small cloche would do the job, or use screens positioned well to break the wind. Make sure the screens are staked well or far away from the plants. If they fall, they could damage the plants more than the wind.

The cabbage white butterfly, as mentioned before, is the fiercest enemy of the cabbage grower. I don't like to use pest control products as I think they interfere too much with nature, although the cabbage white has had me sorely tempted from time to time. The first couple of years I grew cabbages, I never saw any. Then one day, as soon as the cabbages started to grow, the butterflies arrived. If you don't pop into the garden a few times a day you may miss them, so you must check they haven't laid any eggs preferably twice a day. If you are unable to do this for any reason, get someone to do it for you. The eggs are laid on the underside of the leaves to protect the baby caterpillars from birds and the sun. As soon as the eggs hatch, you have the world's hungriest caterpillars to deal with. Within a couple of days these caterpillars will devour your whole plant and move onto the next one, if it hasn't already been eaten. It really is a battle, and although it's not very spiritual I have no qualms about destroying these eating machines. Feed them to your chickens if you have any, or get rid of them any way you can, just get them away from your cabbages!

Cabbage root fly can also be a problem and if you have this pest in your area you may need to use collars on the plants to keep the fly from laying its eggs.

Poly-tunnels and Containers
Generally, cabbages do well in cooler conditions and are not often grown indoors, however, as long as the temperature is fairly cool, you should be able to grow them indoors. Check on the seed packet for any further instructions, or ask at your local garden centre for indoor cabbages. Commercial growers do grow them in poly tunnels and this is probably a good way of growing all year round cabbages. Although it's probably best not to attempt to grow the summer varieties under glass or plastic – the heat would probably be too intense for them. Containers work well with cabbages but they need to be fairly large and deep, and kept well watered.

Storing

Cabbages will store successfully for a few weeks in a dark, dry place. Damp will rot them quickly as they are high in water content. If there are mice in the neighbourhood, stored cabbages can be a prime target. Hanging in nets prevents vermin attacks.

The most popular way to store cabbage is making sauerkraut. This is a process of fermenting the cabbage and storing in jars. The cabbage has to be sliced and mixed with salt, weighed down and left to ferment for a few weeks. Cabbage stores well like this and soups can be made from the fermented cabbage during cold winter months, although the Vitamin C content is about half that of fresh cabbage.

 Celeriac

History

Celeriac originates from wild celery and was grown in Mediterranean areas some 2000 years ago. It didn't become known across Europe until the Middle Ages, and although it is widely grown and eaten in some countries, it still isn't popular in the UK or US.

Celeriac tastes very similar to celery but is not stringy. It can be eaten raw, grated in salads or cooked in stews or soups. A very practical and nutritious vegetable, celeriac is very popular in France and is served regularly with everyday meals.

It has a long growing time and could therefore be considered to be difficult to bring to maturity in a cooler climate. However, there are ways round the problem, and it can be successfully grown in most climates.

Growing Celeriac

Choosing celeriac ~ There are not that many different varieties of celeriac readily available although there are probably about 8 or 9 that will grow in milder climates, so a little searching may prove worthwhile. Ask in your local garden centre for regional favourites.

Prepare the site ~ Celeriac is a heavy feeder and should be grown in rich soil. Dig over at least a month before sowing. The ground should be well-drained but able to hold moisture and the soil shouldn't be too acidic. Generally, celeriac is quite hardy and will grow in most garden soil.

Position ~ Celeriac is a cool weather vegetable but will not tolerate frosts. As the growing season could stretch into the autumn or early winter, it's wise to prepare the site in a fairly sunny position, and avoid any frost pockets or very cold, windy spots in your garden.

Planting celeriac ~ Sow seed inside in seed trays just below the surface of the seed compost, at the end of March or beginning of April. Keep warm and watered for about 3 months until the end of June, or beginning of July. When the seedlings are a few inches high (5 cm.) transplant into another tray to allow the small plants more space to grow. The temperature needs to be kept fairly constant. The celeriac root takes a long time to mature and after about 3 months inside, it will take another 3 months or so in the garden before it's ready to eat.

Around the beginning of July when the plants are looking sturdy enough, plant out in the prepared bed. Allow around 12 in. (30 cm.) of space for each plant and around 2 ft. (60 cm.) between rows. Refer to your seed packet for spacing recommendations.

Caring for celeriac ~ Although celeriac is related to celery and takes a long time to mature, it tends to grow well with little attention. There are few pests that affect the plants.

Celeriac roots will benefit from an organic feed from time to time during the outdoor growing season. As they are heavy feeders this will also help the soil from becoming stripped of too many minerals.

Keep weeded and well watered. The soil should never be allowed to dry out. If celeriac roots are dry, they can become hollow or woody and inedible. A fairly thick mulch during the summer months will help keep the moisture in the ground.

Pull a few roots when they are fairly small for a summer salad treat. Keep pulling celeriac as and when you like. The root will grow fairly big by the time it has fully matured. It can be left in the ground until the cold weather is imminent.

The younger roots will be more tender than the older ones. Pull them all up before the first frost. Some growers say they are frost resistant, but unless your particular variety indicates that it can tolerate frosts, it's just not worth the risk. After that long growing period, you want to make sure you have a good harvest to show for your efforts.

Poly-tunnels and Containers
Greenhouses and poly-tunnels can be used to grow celeriac, but they are a hardy root vegetable and after the first few months of nurturing, the plants can be left outside quite safely until the autumn months. Try a few in your greenhouse or tunnel; some varieties may work better than others. Shallow containers aren't always so practical for root crops but a deep container would be okay.

Storing
Celeriac roots will keep in a cool, dark place for a number of weeks, but make sure they are kept dry. Clean off surplus soil before storing, but don't wash them. Let the roots rest for a day or two, then brush off dry soil and store.

Otherwise, a soup or other recipe can be made with celeriac and frozen quickly and stored in the freezer for many months. Remember to label.

 Onions

History
Onions have been hard to date by archaeologists, but it's generally thought that onions have been eaten since prehistoric times and have been cultivated for at least 5000 years. Onions grew wild and were indigenous to many parts of the

world. They grow in varied soils and nearly every type of climate. The onion can also be stored for food during the colder months of the year.

As well as being a valuable food crop, onions have been used in herbal medicines for many centuries. The ancient Egyptians believed the onion had magical powers and onion bulbs were often buried with the dead to encourage new life. A common preparation, still used today, soothes coughs and alleviates cold symptoms: slice an onion and place in a bowl with a little sugar. Cover and leave overnight. The resulting liquid should be taken first thing in the morning.

Growing Onions

Choosing onions ~ There are regular, everyday, kitchen onions, as well as the very large Spanish onions to choose from. And then there are:

- spring onions
- everlasting onions
- tree onions
- shallots
- red onions
- and plenty more varieties to choose from

Everlasting onions, sometimes referred to as Welsh onions are a good standby crop in the garden as they are ready to use in early spring before other varieties are available. Tree onions grow above the soil on plants and resemble tiny onion trees. Spring onions, although the name indicates a spring harvest, tend to be ready to eat in the early summer months. But this is ideal timing for the early salads and a spring onion or two perfectly compliments early, fresh lettuce leaves. Shallots and red onions are a chef's delight and growing a few of each in your vegetable plot will make for some wonderful culinary delights later on in the year.

Prepare the site ~ Onions like to grow in firm ground so it's better to prepare the site a few months before growing if you can. Dig over and add well-rotted manure or compost. Remove any large stones and perennial weeds.

Position ~ Generally, onions like a sunny position, but check on the growing instructions for your particular variety. They also like a well-drained soil. If your ground is too boggy, the onions will rot very quickly.

Planting onions ~ Regular onions can be planted from seed or 'sets'. Seed should be started earlier in the year to allow enough growing time. Onion seed can sometimes be difficult to get going, and is often taken over by weeds before the onions are established. Young onion plants look exactly like grass and it's almost impossible to tell them apart when the plants are small. Seeds can be started off in trays and then transplanted but aren't always happy to be moved. Read the growing instructions on the seed packets before you buy them.

Spring onions will have to be started from seed. Everlasting onions are better started from someone else's cast-offs. Beg or borrow a clump of everlasting onions from a local grower in the autumn, separate and replant straight away, and by the following spring each onion will have multiplied into a clump of between 6 and 12 usable fresh onions. Use these onions, saving one or two from each clump to replant for next year's crop and replant immediately.

Buying onion sets is by far the easiest way to get a good crop of everyday bulb onions or shallots. Start in early spring, unless the ground is too wet. If the mud sticks, wait a while. Gently firm down the soil before planting. Use a dibber or other hole-producing tool and make holes for the onions leaving around 6–8 in. (15–20 cm.) between each one. Double check your variety for spacing advice. Allow 18 in. between rows so you have enough space to water and weed your plants. Pop each onion or shallot into a hole and cover with soil, leaving a tiny tip of the bulb poking above the soil. Firm down the soil around each onion set. It's a good idea to fix a net or some protection over the onions until they start growing, as birds like to pull them out of the ground. When you've finished planting, water well.

Japanese or tree onions are normally planted at the end of the summer, but these varieties have their own unique growing criteria so check on the growing instructions before you plant.

Caring for onions ~ Onions can be attacked by the 'onion fly'. A good way to prevent this happening is to alternate the rows with carrots. Carrots repel the onion fly and onions repel the carrot fly, so everyone's happy! Onion fly only seems to attack onions grown from seed, not those grown from sets. If onion fly is a problem in your area then you may find it better to just grow onion sets.

If the onions do get a bug or virus, use an organic solution to cure the problem. Your local garden centre should have organic products available. Make sure the ground doesn't dry out during hot weather; watering regularly will ensure good growth. Although onions do like to be kept well watered in the summer months, don't be tempted to mulch to keep moisture in the ground; the onions will rot. They need fresh air and well-drained soil.

Onions are fairly hardy and were growing wild amongst many other plants for centuries. For this reason many gardeners will insist that onions will grow and develop well in a bed of weeds. But personally I've always found I get a much better crop if I give the onions some space to breathe. It is advisable to keep weed-free as much as possible.

When the leaves start to go brown they are almost ready to harvest. Fold down the leaves carefully so as not to snap them and leave for a few more days. Sometimes onions will go to seed. They send up a very hard stem and produce a flower. Some growers snap this off; others leave it or fold it down if possible. I found if I snap the stem off and leave the onion in the ground for another week or two, it will be fine. The onions that go to seed don't store as well and should be used straight away. The centre will probably be woody and inedible, but just cut that part out before using. Pull up the onions on a sunny day and lay on the soil to dry for a couple of hours in the sun, turning occasionally.

Poly-tunnels and Containers
Onions can be planted in deep containers quite successfully, just make sure the soil doesn't dry out. They are not really very compatible with greenhouse or poly-tunnel growing but a few of the newer varieties around may be good to try.

Storing

Onions will store for a number of months if kept in a dry area; if the climate isn't too damp, they can be strung and kept in a shed or barn. After you've pulled the onions and dried them in the sun for a few hours, bring them indoors and store in boxes, or plait into lengths, and hang from the ceiling. Wait until the leaves are dry or they may rot, and try to plait them so that the onions don't press against each other. Stored properly, onions will last for many months. A string of onions in the kitchen is just as useful as a string of garlic, and makes the whole kitchen look very professional.

Potatoes

History

Potatoes are so common in the western diet; we imagine they have been part of the human diet forever. But although evidence suggests potatoes were used around 500BC, the potato had a bad reputation for many centuries and was considered an evil vegetable by a number of civilisations. The leaves and stems of the potato plant are poisonous and it was probably because of this and the fact that the weird, lumpy looking, unattractive tuber didn't appear to be edible that gave the potato a bad name. Thank goodness we now know better! It took a few hundred years and many persistent voyagers to get the potato introduced to the dinner table of the western world. Of course the Irish potato famine is probably one of the most famous potato stories, and the Irish people do have many myths and legends attached to the potato.

Growing Potatoes

Choosing potatoes ~ There are many different varieties of seed potato to choose from. Some will provide you with a softer potato that is better for mashing, and others will be a harder type used in potato salads for example. Your garden centre will stock the best potatoes for your region and it's a nice idea to plant some of each if you have the space available. Seed potatoes should be no bigger than an egg when you buy them.

Prepare the site ~ Our best ever potato harvest was a result of good preparation, and a little luck with the weather. We dug, trenched and laid comfrey leaves in the bottom of the trench. Then we scattered a little earth back on top of the comfrey and placed our potatoes on top. The comfrey feeds the roots of the plant as it grows. This method resulted in a wonderful crop of potatoes.

Position ~ Potatoes can be very hardy but will produce a greater crop if grown in a sunny spot. Don't plant near tomatoes – they are of the same family of plants and will be more prone to getting blight diseases if too close.

Sowing potatoes ~ Before sowing, potatoes need to 'sprout'. Spread the potatoes out in a shallow cardboard box, or similar container, and leave in a dry, airy place for a couple of weeks. Avoid direct sunlight. After a couple of weeks, there should be a few sprouts on each potato and they are ready to plant.

The traditional method: Many gardeners will tell you that potatoes help break up the soil, and should be the first crop on a previously un-worked piece of land. And it does work. We filled our new plot with potato seed and the following year the soil was much easier to work. The downside? A smaller harvest. While we did have lots of delicious potatoes, subsequent years have proved that the harvest tends to be greater if the soil is prepared before sowing.

Dig your ground and create a trench about 6–8 in. deep. Place your potato seed carefully along the line, about 12 in. apart. Cover seed carefully by hand and rake gently over the ground when trenches are filled. Water if weather is dry and wait patiently for a couple of weeks. Keep an eye on your patch and remove any weeds as they appear. After 2–3 weeks, you will see small, bushy-looking plants popping up in the row.

Caring for potatoes ~ When the plants are around 8 in. high, gently pull the soil up and over the plants leaving a couple of centimetres showing. Use a rake, Dutch hoe or similar tool. The row should now be raised along it's whole length by about 6–8 in. Don't take these measurements too literally. You will feel what is right for your plot as you work it.

After a few more weeks, the whole 'earthing up' process needs to be repeated. The reason for this is that the potatoes will grow inside the mound you have created. If potatoes aren't covered properly when growing, they go green and become poisonous.

By now, you should have a fair sized mound and the plants will be growing well. Water every day if weather is dry and keep free of weeds. 'Earth up' your plants once more about 2–3 weeks later. Then leave them alone. Now spring should be dissolving into summer and you won't want to be doing too much heavy work in the garden. As the weather becomes drier, remember to water your potato plot well. Potatoes need a lot of water to fully develop.

Sowing potatoes – with less back work: Growing potatoes in the traditional way is labour intensive, and over the years new methods have been tried and tested to grow healthy crops of potatoes.

Raised beds – Creating narrow strips of land to grow your crops is becoming more and more popular. The theory is that you dig less, and also, because you don't ever walk onto your plot, the soil will not be compacted and lose it's natural structure. Make your beds less than a metre wide, so that you can comfortably reach to the middle of the bed from either side. Once dug, you mustn't step onto the prepared soil.

Use a fence post or any 'hole-making' implement and make holes for your potatoes along the bed. Give each seed about 12 in. all around. Plant in a couple of rows, staggered to keep the spacing right. Place seed in holes and cover.

Sowing potatoes in this way means you will not need to 'earth up' as they grow. However, when we tried this method, we found that the plants were much more vulnerable to wind, as they tended to grow more straggly than bushy. The crop was good though.

Barrels – If space is limited, potatoes can be grown in containers. In early spring plant a few potatoes in a couple of old car tyres. Fill a tyre with prepared soil (any well-rotted compost or soil from another part of your garden will do, as long as it is broken up well and all weeds removed). Place a few early variety potatoes into the tyre – around 3–6 depending on the size of your tyre. If the weather is cold, place a small sheet of clear plastic over the tyre and tuck in to keep the plants cosy during the cold nights. Remove during the day for light and air.

Problems ~ Potatoes are subject to a number of diseases, the most prevalent of which is 'blight'. If you find you have the disease, cut down the foliage of the plant (burn the diseased plant if you can) and the potatoes will continue to grow for a few more weeks. However, when you do get a serious blight attack, there is little you can do, except cry perhaps. Sowing potatoes isn't always easy. There are ways of preventing the fungus attack. Many gardeners swear by 'Bordeaux mixture'. The liquid is sprayed onto the foliage of the potato plants a number of times during the growth period. Muggy weather encourages the blight fungus so keep a careful eye on your crop during warm and damp weather conditions.

The harvest ~ As soon as a potato plant has flowers, the tiny potatoes under the soil start swelling. If you gently push away the soil from the bottom of a plant, you can pick a few early new potatoes. Go on you deserve it! When the foliage has completely died back, your potato crop is ready to harvest. Use a fork or spade and dig up your plants from the outside of the mound. Don't dig straight through the middle, or you may damage some of your valuable crop. Lay the potatoes out to dry in the sun for a few hours, turning occasionally. Don't leave too long as sunlight will turn your potatoes green, and make them inedible.

Poly-tunnels and Containers
Early potatoes can be grown in poly-tunnels and under cloches. But later varieties benefit from fresh air and should be grown outside wherever possible.

Storing
There are a variety of styles of potato storage systems in use, or make your own. Collect fruit cartons (shallow cardboard boxes) with air holes. Place your potatoes in single layers in the boxes and store in a cool, dry, dark place. They should keep well for a few months. Remember that potatoes have a high water content and are very vulnerable to frosts. An overnight frost will rot a whole crop of potatoes in a cold barn or shed. Keep an eye on the temperature, and bring the potatoes in if you need to.

Chapter Eight

Growing Plants Rich in Vitamin C

Blackcurrants, Peppers, Strawberries, Tomatoes

Blackcurrants

History

Blackcurrants are an ancient fruit and were probably picked from wild plants thousands of years ago. Blackcurrants have been used medicinally since the middle ages to treat many different health problems; although it wasn't until the 19th to 20th centuries we started to understand the full nutritional value of blackcurrants. They are packed full of vitamins and minerals and are probably one of the best garden fruits to grow.

During World War II, it was very difficult to find sources of vitamin C in the UK; the government encouraged blackcurrants to be grown, as they have one of the highest levels of vitamin C of any fruit. Consequently the whole of the blackcurrant crop in the UK was made into cordials and British children grew up on the healthy juice. Blackcurrant juice is still an incredibly popular drink in the UK and across the world.

Growing blackcurrants

Choosing blackcurrants ~ There are a number of new hybrid varieties of blackcurrants that produce fruits as large as grapes. They are also sweeter and need less sugar added.

There are many different varieties of blackcurrant and your local garden centre may stock the most compatible plants for your region.

Blackcurrants can also be started by pushing a cut off branch from an old plant into the ground. Not all canes will grow so it's worth growing quite a number of them. If they are still going after the first year, dig up gently and transplant to your chosen site.

Prepare the site ~ Blackcurrants are generally a very hardy crop and will grow in more or less any soil type.

To get the best crops, a little preparation is needed. Dig the ground over and remove any perennial weeds and non-organic debris. Dig in some well-rotted manure or compost. The ground should be moist but well-drained. Blackcurrants won't do well in very dry or waterlogged ground.

Position ~ Blackcurrants like full sun but will tolerate a little shade if they have to.

Planting blackcurrants ~ Plant blackcurrant bushes from early winter to early spring, anytime when it's not too cold or wet. Dig a hole a bit bigger than the root structure and a little deeper. Tease out the roots gently and plant. Firm the soil around each plant. They should be spaced about 6 ft. (2 metres) apart.

It's advisable to prune the plant straight away, by cutting all branches down to around the second bud up from the ground. This seems a bit extreme but it will encourage the roots to grow as well as sending up more branches – more branches mean more fruit! Check on the planting recommendations on your variety before you do this though.

Caring for blackcurrants ~ Water blackcurrants regularly and don't let the ground dry out. Mulching helps to retain water, and if you mulch with good garden compost, you'll feed the plants at the same time. Mulching also helps to prevent weeds taking over.

Apart from the first year, blackcurrant bushes should be pruned every winter. Leave to settle in the first year but from the second winter on, prune carefully. Take about 20% out of the middle of the plant and cut away any dead wood or branches that are twisted together or crossing over each other. Use a sharp pair of secateurs (pruning shears) to do this so you don't damage the remaining wood by tearing it.

It's also advisable to take a little wood from the outside of the plant, but not too much. You may have pruning instructions for your particular variety of blackcurrant. Read these first before you start snipping. New hybrid varieties could have different requirements.

Blackcurrants should be picked on a dry day – the fruit will deteriorate much quicker if wet or damp when picked.

Poly-tunnels and Containers

Blackcurrant bushes are really an outdoor crop and unless you live in a particularly difficult growing region, for example very close to the sea or the North Pole, it's probably best to stick with outdoor growing.

The same applies to containers. You may possibly be able to get some fruit from a container grown blackcurrant but it's unlikely the plant will thrive if root growth is restricted in any way.

Storing

Traditionally blackcurrants have been made into jellies and jams and this is an ideal way to store them almost indefinitely. Otherwise, pies, tarts and other desserts can be made, frozen quickly and stored in the freezer for several months. Remember to label the container. Check the recipe section in Chapter Fifteen for other ideas.

You can also make your own blackcurrant juice and freeze or bottle. If you don't use preserving sugar the bottled juice will have to be consumed fairly quickly. Keep in the fridge for a longer shelf life.

Fresh blackcurrants will keep fairly well for five or six days in the fridge but don't wash them before putting in the fridge. The new hybrid varieties produce sweet fruits and it's unlikely that you'll be able to grow enough to store as they will be so easy to pick and eat!

Peppers

History

There is archaeological evidence of wild peppers being cultivated for human consumption as far back as 5000 BC. Chilli peppers were believed to have originated in India for many centuries but they actually came from South America. The pepper became more widely known and used after Columbus discovered it in the 16th century. By the late 16th century, peppers were used in all regions of the world, especially in Europe and India.

Peppers come in so many varieties, shapes and sizes it would be impossible to list them all. But for the average gardener and consumer, we can grow and eat the types that are compatible with the local climate. There are two different species: the chili pepper and the sweet pepper. Some chili peppers are so spicy they are almost impossible to eat for those with an undeveloped palate for such tastes. However, the sweet pepper is usually acceptable for all palates; even young children enjoy the texture and colours of sweet peppers.

Growing Peppers

Choosing peppers ~ There are many varieties of peppers, whether you want to grow the sweet or spicy varieties, and it's best to browse through a catalogue or visit your local garden centre to see what they have on offer. Normally, the seeds or plants sold in your region will be compatible with your climate. However, double check on the growing instructions as some may be better grown in a cloche, greenhouse or poly-tunnel.

Sweet peppers are said to be mature when red or even black, but the colour of the harvested fruit is often dependant on the variety. I have grown green sweet peppers for many years and none have ever reached the 'red' stage without rotting first. This development depends on the length of the growing season in your region. Try a couple of different varieties if you haven't grown them before. Take a few notes on their growing time, ease of care and how you like the taste.

If you like to cook Mexican or other spicy foods, grow a few hot chili peppers. The plants are very attractive even if the peppers are too hot for you. I found hot chili peppers nearly always had time to turn red before harvesting. There is a theory that hot peppers increase the metabolism.

Prepare the site ~ Dig in some well-rotted manure or compost as early as you can in the year. Or if you are growing in containers, get them ready and keep the soil weed-free and fairly fine in texture. Peppers, as with many other plants, don't like waterlogged soil. The roots and stem will rot very quickly in boggy conditions. The soil should be well-drained. Choose a bright spot but if you can only plant your peppers in direct sunlight, you may have to shade them during the hottest part of the day and they will certainly need lots of watering.

Position ~ Don't plant your peppers in soil that grew potatoes or tomatoes the previous year. They belong to the same plant family and could pick up diseases in the soil. To avoid cross-pollination keep sweet peppers and hot peppers away from each other.

Peppers are originally a tropical plant and like to grow in warm soil. They prefer a sunny spot but long periods in direct sunlight can damage the flowers and leaves. They like the morning sun, and grow very well in containers near the house.

Sowing peppers ~ Start your peppers off fairly late in the spring, even though it's tempting to get them going early. I've always found the small plants' growth was restricted by cold temperatures and although those plants may well reach full maturity, they don't tend to produce so much fruit.

Pepper plants are often available to buy ready for planting out – these plants are usually started off in poly-tunnels or protected areas. Don't be fooled into thinking they are probably frost hardy or even ready to be put out in your garden – keep an eye on the weather and watch when other growers put their peppers out. Otherwise, do it yourself and start with seeds. Plant seed in shallow trays of seed compost and keep moist and well-drained. Don't allow the roots of the new pepper plants to sit in water.

When the plants are a few inches (6 cm.) tall and have 3 or 4 true leaves, re-pot them into separate containers ready for planting out in the garden later. Ordinary flower pots or any plastic pots will do, as long as they are well-drained. There are a number of pots on the market that are planted along with the plant. These pots decompose naturally, and also let you handle the plants without fear of damaging the roots. Your local garden centre will probably have some.

Once you've re-potted your pepper plants, keep warm and watered and wait for the best day to plant outside. Check your local growing guides and regional zones for exact timing. Asking other local gardeners will give you a good idea. Mostly use your own instinct. It's your garden, live with nature for a while and you'll soon 'just know' when the time is right!

Many people garden according to the moon phase. They believe you should plant out during the days when the moon starts to wane. The gravitational downward pull helps to establish a good root structure. You should definitely wait until all danger of a frost has passed.

Caring for peppers ~ Allow around 45cm. in each direction for the plants to grow.

Keep a close eye on your plants when you first put them out. Slugs love young plants, and will eat through the stems of your seedlings given half a chance. Crushed eggshells placed around the plants will deter slugs and snails. Attracting frogs helps to keep slugs under control as well.

Water your peppers regularly but make sure they don't get waterlogged. Don't let the weeds take over in the early weeks. As the plants get bigger they create their own micro-climate. A sweet pepper patch looks like a mini rain forest when it gets going! The leaves protect the fruits and the shade prevents the weeds coming up. Hot chili peppers normally produce smaller leaves and generally less foliage so there may be a little more weeding to do.

Other than watering, especially in dry weather, peppers more or less look after themselves. However, if your peppers are exposed to long periods of direct sunlight, they may suffer. Watch out for this and protect the plants during the hottest part of the day by draping a cover over the pepper patch. A very lightweight sheet of material or a special gardening cover can be used. Remember to remove it when the direct light isn't so intense to allow the plants to fully develop.

If you live in a region with a long growing season, your peppers may mature to a full red colour and should be allowed to do so. Otherwise, picking your peppers at the green stage is perfectly acceptable. Many people prefer the texture of the green pepper as it tends to be slightly crispier and sharper in taste.

When the fruits are ready to pick, cut the stalk with a sharp knife to avoid damaging the rest of the plant. Make sure all peppers are harvested before the first frost.

Poly-tunnels and Containers

Peppers, sweet or hot, can be grown inside, in a light, airy part of the house, conservatory or greenhouse.

They can also be grown very successfully in containers, large pots or even window boxes. Keep the soil in containers and pots moist and cover or move into the shade during the hottest part of the day. Don't leave pots in the shade as the fruits won't develop well.

Storing

Peppers will keep for up to a couple of weeks in the salad compartment of the fridge or a cold place. It's possible to freeze them, but as they have a high water content they don't keep their nice, crisp texture. Use them in a ratatouille or other dish and freeze the whole meal. (See Chapter Fifteen for recipe ideas.) Alternatively, peppers can be bottled (canned) and stored for many months, although they do lose some of their bright, green colour in the processing.

Hot peppers can be dried and kept for up to a year, maybe longer. Dry them whole in the sun or over a hot stove for a few days and store in a sealed jar. Be careful when handling hot chili peppers – they can cause irritation of the skin. Don't touch your eyes directly after handling them.

Strawberries

History

Wild strawberries have grown over large parts of the world for thousands of years but they are not as sweet as the cultivated strawberry we enjoy today. The red, sweet strawberry was first cultivated around the 16th century and symbolised love, purity and all things sweet for many years. In fact it was said at one time that if you broke a heart-shaped strawberry in half and both you and your sweetheart ate a half, you would fall deeply in love.

Strawberries are also reputed to have healing powers, and apart from being high in vitamin C content, they do contain many vitamins and minerals beneficial to the human body. They have been said to heal all kinds of ailments including kidney disorders and throat infections. The leaves of the strawberry plant are also beneficial and strawberry tea can be bought readily in most health food shops and supermarkets.

Growing Strawberries

Choosing strawberries ~ There are quite a number of different varieties to choose from, including seasonal varieties. Some fruit in early summer and some types fruit much later in the year. Your local garden centre will stock the best regional varieties.

Choose a variety that produces lots of fruit if you have children in the house, as they do tend to go and pick them when you're not looking!

Don't be tempted to use a wild plant to get your strawberry patch going. Wild strawberries are not as sweet as hybrids and often don't even go red. They produce very small fruits that are barely edible.

Another way of starting your strawberry patch is to beg baby plants from local growers. When the plants throw out runners they produce new plants, and these can get discarded if there are too many. If you know a friendly strawberry grower, ask them to save you some.

Prepare the site ~ Don't use ground where tomatoes, potatoes or peppers have been grown in recent years. These vegetables can leave a virus in the ground that will seriously damage strawberry plants.

Dig over the ground in the autumn before spring planting and incorporate well-rotted manure or compost. Remove any non-organic debris as well as perennial weeds. Cover the ground for the winter months and remove covering a week or so before you plant the strawberries.

Strawberries can get straggly and constructing a purpose built strawberry bed will be helpful. Choose a sunny spot and stake off a square for the bed. Make a border of wood, rocks, bricks, or anything non-metallic so as to raise the bed slightly. Pour a layer of good compost on top of the freshly dug and prepared soil. Cover and leave until the spring planting.

Position ~ Strawberries like a sunny spot and will produce the best fruits when planted in full sun.

Planting strawberries ~ Each strawberry plant should be put in the ground so that the roots are just covered with soil, but not the 'crown'. Allow around 12 in. (30cm) of space between plants and around 18 in. (45 cm.) between rows. This is a general estimate. It's a good idea to check on the planting instructions when you buy your strawberries as varieties will vary in size and growing requirements. Water the plants well.

Caring for strawberries ~ Although strawberries are one of the most popular fruits to grow in the home garden, there are all kinds of different systems and plenty of conflicting advice. The following notes are a general overview to caring for your strawberries but it's always a good idea to go with your instincts as well as talking to local growers.

Water strawberry plants regularly and keep weed free. Mulch during the hot summer months to help keep moisture in the ground. When the fruits start growing, they are vulnerable to slug attacks and can become damaged if laying on wet soil. Mulching with a fine dry straw solves both these problems. Strawberries are also very attractive to birds, and you should cover with a net if possible. Use a very fine netting so that the birds don't get their wings tangled.

Some growers believe you should pick off all the flowers in the first year so that the plants produce more fruit in subsequent years.

Strawberry plants can be damaged by frost and extreme cold weather and a cloche during early spring and winter will help. There are covers available for plant protection if building a cloche doesn't work for you.

During the growing season, the 'mother' plant will send off runners and produce baby plants at the end of each one. These will plant themselves if they can, otherwise you can gently push them into the soil. These baby plants can be left to grow in following years or removed and replanted in a new bed at the end of the season.

I like to keep my strawberry bed fairly tidy and remove the new plants. The original plants produce more fruit without the runners attached. Read the growing instructions when you buy your plants or ask local growers what they do. Different varieties will respond in different ways.

Strawberry beds should be renewed every three years. If you remove baby plants at the end of the year, these plants can be used to start off a new patch. With enough space in the garden, you can rotate three beds quite successfully.

Poly-tunnels and Containers
Strawberries are perfect to grow in containers and purpose made strawberry barrels are readily available. They can be grown in virtually any container and will thrive if kept well watered. Strawberries will also grow in greenhouses and poly-tunnels successfully.

Storing
The fresh fruit will only keep for a few days but strawberries can be frozen, although they change their texture quite dramatically. They will freeze more successfully if frozen when already incorporated in a baked dish, such as a strawberry tart. The most traditional way of storing strawberries is by making jam.

Tomatoes

History

The tomato is known to have been grown as a food crop by the Incan civilisation around 1000 AD, but was believed to be poisonous by many other cultures across the world. In the mid 1500s, Italians grew tomatoes as an ornamental plant. Over the next few hundred years, tomatoes travelled throughout Europe and were known for their ornamental flowers, even as a strong aphrodisiac, but were nearly always grown for decorative purposes.

In the early 19th century, businessmen realised the great potential the tomato had in the marketplace and reclassified it as a vegetable rather than a fruit; vegetables had more freedom in the marketplace than fruit. This was an excellent move for the savvy businessman of the time who ate tomatoes in public places to prove their safety and goodness.

The earliest recorded tomato ketchup recipe was in 1818.

Growing Tomatoes

Choosing tomatoes ~ There are hundreds of varieties of tomatoes and browsing through seed packets and making a sensible decision can take the best part of an afternoon if you're not careful!

There are four main types of tomato:

The regular family tomato – used in all salads, cooked dishes and as a garnish on an elegant buffet. Larger tomatoes can be stuffed and served as a main meal. If you decide to start your tomato garden using ready grown plants, you will find the regular family tomato is one of the more popular types available.

Cherry Tomatoes – decorative, slightly sweet and always a favourite with the kids. Cherry tomatoes come in all sorts of shapes and colours, and even sizes. Some are very small, while others are a regular 'cherry' size. Cut regular cherry tomatoes in half and add them to a green salad. They are a very popular garden variety and nurseries are beginning to stock the plants as well as the regular varieties.

Plum Tomatoes – normally available in cans, the plum tomato isn't that popular as a garden plant. I grew yellow plum tomatoes for a few years. They were hardly bigger than a cherry tomato and so popular it was hard to keep any on the plant. Exactly the kind of veggie you can pop in your mouth while strolling round the garden! The larger red plum tomatoes are fun to grow and it's always worth experimenting if you have the space.

Beefsteak Tomatoes – Beefsteak is a general name for the very large, chunky tomatoes and there are many varieties. Large tomatoes are great for sandwiches; they slice easily and go a long way. When they get too soft for slicing, beefsteak tomatoes can be successfully used in cooking. Remove any solid core, peel and throw the rest in the pot. Beefsteak tomatoes can also be stuffed and baked.

With all the tomatoes available how do you choose? Here are a few pointers and questions to help you decide:

- Do you already have any family favourites?
- How do you usually enjoy your tomatoes?
- How would you like to enjoy your tomatoes?
- Do you have kids in the house?
- Is space a problem?
- How many different types do you want to grow?

If you can, check out a catalogue or two before you head off to the garden centre. Online seed stores are also a good place to start. They often provide numerous varieties with photographs and growing tips.

Prepare the site ~ Make sure the site is well-drained and in a sunny position. Although tomatoes will grow in sub-standard soil, the plants will not yield a heavy crop and it's far better to grow them in good quality soil. Get your soil analysed if you think it necessary, or just dig in lots of well-rotted manure or compost in the autumn/winter months.

In spring, dig over well, and till the earth until it is fairly fine. Remove any weeds, and keep removing them until you are ready to plant out your tomatoes. If the weeding becomes a chore, consider covering the area with black plastic or old cardboard, anything that will not contaminate the soil underneath. If the light doesn't get to the soil, the weeds don't grow.

Remove the covering a week or so before planting to give the soil time to breathe.

Position ~ Most sowing instructions will have you planting your tomatoes in rows, some a half metre apart in rows 2 metres apart, etc; however, from experience I know that this doesn't always work well. Tomatoes are very susceptible to blight viruses, and if you have all the tomatoes lined up, the virus invades every single plant. Beating these viruses and still avoiding chemical remedies is possible – just scatter your plants around the garden. Check on the packet for distances so you know roughly how big your plants will get.

Planting your tomatoes all over the garden may seem odd, but get creative. You could plant 2 or 3 in a row at the end of one small plot, a couple in the flower beds, one or two in the herbs, a line of five against a fence. Get imaginative and try lots of ideas. Go for sunny spots and avoid windy locations. Finding homes for two or three dozen tomato plants will be a lot easier than you think.

Sowing tomatoes ~ You have the choice of growing tomatoes from ready starter plants or from seed. There isn't always as much variety when buying the plants, but if you're looking for a fast and easy family type tomato, buying plants is the best choice.

If you're buying ready starter plants from the nursery, late spring will be the best planting time. Always plant after the last possible frost. This date varies from region to region. In the UK, mid-May is a good time to be planting out tomatoes. If you are growing the plants in a greenhouse, buy them as soon as they are in the shop and plant under glass straight away. Water well.

Starting from seed is another story!

Plant the seeds quite early because you want to be able to plant them out in late spring to get a full growing season and a good crop. Start about eight weeks before the last frost. You'll need somewhere warm to keep them; a greenhouse, conservatory or a sunny windowsill.

Prepare a seed tray with good quality seed potting soil. Sow your seeds and moisten the soil with a gentle watering system; a small water sprayer is ideal. Put markers in each tray with the name of the variety and the date the seeds were planted. It's always good to know how long seeds take to germinate, for next time. A good reason to keep a gardening journal. It will be a few weeks until your plants are ready to pot, and the soil should be kept fairly warm and moist during this time. Make sure your seed trays are well-drained.

Potting ~ When your tomato plants are 20–30 cm. high, they will need re-potting. Prepare individual pots for this. You can use black plastic pots you've used before, yoghurt pots, or specialist trays of individual pots that can be planted straight into the ground. The choice is yours — go with your budget. The most important thing is making sure the drainage is good. Punch holes in the base of your pots if needed, and put a little gravel in the bottom of each one before filling with potting soil.

Half fill the pots with potting soil or use your own mix. It has to be quite fine, though. Put through a sieve before using. Water the plants and then carefully ease them out of the seed tray to avoid damage. Handle by the stem as much as possible, and avoid contact with the roots.

Place each tomato plant into it's own pot and fill with soil to the top. Firm down the plant and add a little more soil if needed. Sink the whole pot up to the rim in a bowl of water (not too cold). Remove immediately and leave to drain in a warm, sunny place. You may need to add a little more soil when the level has dropped.

Look after your pots. Water regularly and keep them warm for another month or so, and they should be ready to plant out in late spring / early summer.

How many? ~ For a seasonal crop to feed a family of four and a few extras, you should plant about 6 tomato plants. If you want to freeze some for the winter months, consider planting 2 or 3 more plants. Tomato plants do take up some space, so finding places for 40 or 50 plants may not be feasible. Don't try and grow all the plants you take from the seed trays — you may have hundreds. Throw the weaker plants away.

Planting out ~ You need a stake for each plant. Buy special tomato support canes from your local garden centre or if you have access to large numbers of straight branches or off-cuts that are big enough, use them.

Make sure your ground is prepared (weed-free, well dug, hoed, raked etc.) Dig a hole a little larger than the pot holding your tomato. Place stake or cane in the ground right next to the hole and make sure it's very firm. Dunk the pot in water and let it drain for a few seconds then ease the tomato plant gently from the pot. Tease the roots out carefully and place in prepared hole. Fill with fine soil and firm down the plant with both hands. Water well.

Using a natural garden string, make a loose tie around the plant and stake. This will protect the young plant from any high winds.

Voila! Plants are in. Now treat yourself to a cup of tea and consider growing flowers in your veggie patch. I've always allowed nasturtiums to wander freely in the garden, and they make a great companion plant to tomatoes because they attract all the good insects. The same with marigolds. And the best part is that both nasturtiums and marigolds are edible plants!

Caring for tomatoes ~ Tomatoes do need a little looking after. Keep an eye on them and make sure they get enough water. Tomato skins tend to split when they are thirsty.

After a couple of weeks, you can feed the plants, and every couple of weeks after that. Use a comfrey tonic or organic feed.

As the tomato plants grow, tie another loop of twine to the stakes, higher up. Don't let them droop. The stems will break and the plant will die.

When your tomato plants start to grow, they will develop little branches between a branch and the main stem, rather like an armpit growing an extra little arm! Pick these out when you see them. Leaving them will give you a lovely bushy plant but very little fruit. By picking them out, you encourage the main branches to produce more fruit. You should wear gloves to protect your skin when picking out. Tomato plants stain the skin and some people are allergic.

Poly-tunnels and Container

Tomatoes can be very successfully grown in a greenhouse, conservatory or even a good sunny windowsill. Tomatoes will thrive under lights and much of the world's tomato-growing industry uses hydroponic systems. If you are growing tomatoes under lights, try a few different varieties.

Tomatoes need the right nutrients and plenty of water and warmth to thrive. Given these conditions, the plant will reward you with one of the best sources of vitamin C known to humankind.

Storing

Storing tomatoes in your refrigerator is fine, although some experts say a tomato should never be refrigerated or it will turn mushy. If you need to ripen them off a little, keep them at room temperature in a paper bag for a few days. Sometimes your tomato harvest will exceed your wildest expectations and you won't know what to do with them all!

The simplest way of keeping tomatoes is by making a puree and freezing in suitable containers. There is also the possibility of sun drying, if you have the climate. Cut tomatoes in half, sprinkle a little fine sea salt over them and spread out on a tray in the sun for up to a couple of weeks. Cover with a net cover. Don't let it touch the tomatoes and don't let the tomatoes touch each other. Bring whole tray in every night and put out again in the morning. You really have to be able to rely on at least 4 days of full sunshine to get this to work properly. Remove the tomatoes from the trays when they are fully dried. The smaller ones will dry faster. Check every evening and remove the fully dried tomatoes storing them in sealable plastic bags.

If you don't have the climate to sun dry, oven drying will produce very similar results. Cut tomatoes in half and sprinkle with a little fine sea salt. Place on a metal rack, and make sure the tomatoes aren't touching each other. Place rack in a very cool oven (275F, 140C or gas mark 1) for at least 6–8 hours, maybe longer depending on the size of your tomatoes. If 6–8 hours sounds like a crazy amount of time to have the oven on, make the most of it, and stick a casserole in for dinner, and a rice pudding for dessert. Take the tomatoes out of the oven as soon as they dry and cool thoroughly. Store in sealable plastic bags.

You could also sprinkle a few finely chopped herbs on the tomatoes before you start the drying process. Basil is the perfect herb to enhance the flavour of tomatoes, but other herbs and spices will produce their own unique flavour. Experiment a little. Try a very mild curry spice or fresh, finely chopped coriander.

Green Tomato Note
Do you still have unripened or green tomatoes on your plants at the end of the season? When autumn has set in, and your remaining tomatoes aren't going to ripen anymore, try using them in some green tomato recipes, such as pickles and chutneys.

Chapter Nine

Growing Plants Rich in Vitamin E

Asparagus, Dandelion Greens, Raspberries, Sunflower Seeds

sparagus

History

Asparagus has long been considered to be the food of kings and for many years was said to be a 'luxury' crop and even sneered at in a practical everyday garden. But asparagus must be one of the most nutritious and practical vegetables on the planet.

It has been documented as far back as Roman times and it seems the Romans taught others how to grow asparagus. It has also cropped up in ancient Egyptian writings. Europeans really caught on to growing asparagus around the 16th century and the first colonists of America took the seed with them. Asparagus grows in many diverse areas of the globe, although it is indigenous to coastal areas with a sandy soil, and thrives with seaweed fertilisers. It has been considered a medicinal as well as a delicious food.

Growing Asparagus

Choosing asparagus ~ Growing asparagus from seed is time consuming and it will probably be close to five years before you harvest your first crop. Asparagus spears shouldn't be cut from plants less than three years old, so if you buy three year old crowns you can enjoy your first meal of asparagus the following year.

If you can buy male plants, you will find they produce better crops than female plants. Female plants have to produce extra energy to develop seeds and therefore they produce less asparagus stems. I have grown female plants, collected the seed and grown fully mature plants from these seeds. It is worth the effort but only if you have space and the inclination to look after your plants for a number of years before they produce a crop for you.

Prepare the site ~ Asparagus doesn't get moved once planted so you need to find a site that you can leave to your asparagus for the foreseeable future. For this reason it's best to prepare well.

Growing asparagus in soil with a ph of 6.5 to 7.5 is preferred. It's worth testing your soil before planting. If all elements are in order, asparagus will keep on producing spears for 15 years or more. Dig the soil deeply and work to a fine consistency. Mix in sand and any organic matter you need to make up the ph. Rotted seaweed and fish meal are good fertilisers for asparagus. Dig in whatever you have available before planting. The land must be well-drained. Asparagus, like most garden vegetables, will not tolerate wet feet, and the roots will rot quickly if the soil is water-logged

Position ~ Asparagus thrives in full sun. Prepare your site in a sunny area but make sure the plants won't shade other plants. Usually the northern side of your garden works best for this. When you stop cutting your asparagus for the year, the plants will get quite tall, producing attractive fern-like foliage.

Planting asparagus ~ Plant the spider-like crowns 5–6 in. deep, firm the soil and cover with a layer of mixed sand and soil. Sand helps to deter slugs from the young plants. Don't compact the soil. Space the crowns about 12–18 in. (30–45 cm.) apart in each row. Rows should be at least 2 feet apart (60 cm.). Water well. Warm moist soil is the best medium for growing asparagus although it can be drought resistant. Always ensure the soil is well-drained.

Caring for asparagus ~ After planting, the asparagus spears should start to show through the surface of the soil in about a week or two. DON'T CUT spears in the first year of growing. Keep weed-free throughout the growing year. Allow the ferns to die back on their own, and remove in early spring the following year. Dead stalks can be sharp, protect your hands with thick gloves.

In subsequent years, cut the ferns back in the autumn or when they start to die. Then cover the bed with seaweed or other organic matter. Remove any un-rotted material very early in spring and add more soil and sand to raise the bed. The crowns get bigger every year and the bed will need raising accordingly.

In early spring, asparagus crowns can be gently dug out of the ground, divided and replanted to produce more plants. This is probably best done after your first crops and only when the plants are looking large or getting too close together.

Watch for asparagus beetle in late summer and autumn. The beetle feeds on the ferns and the crop is reduced the following year so get rid of them. It's best to use an organic product or pick them off as they arrive.

Harvesting ~ Cut the asparagus spears when they are 7–9 in. long. Some asparagus growers cut the spears just under the surface of the soil. Others believe the roots can be damaged by cutting too low. The best way is to cut as close to the surface of the soil as possible using a sharp knife. Cut in the morning and wash in ice-cold water to remove any heat in the spears or they go limp.

Poly-tunnels and Containers

Asparagus can be grown in greenhouses and poly-tunnels and with a little care and attention the plants can produce edible spears almost all year.

Containers aren't very practical for asparagus as the crowns get larger every year. They prefer to have space for their roots which grow very long and thick.

Storing

Asparagus can be frozen, bottled (canned) or even dried but is always preferable to eat it fresh if you can. Freezing a dish made with asparagus works well. Make asparagus soup or any other favourite recipe, put into suitable containers and freeze quickly. Label and store in the freezer. It will keep for several months.

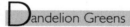
Dandelion Greens

History

Dandelions have been used for many centuries as a healing herb and a delicious food. The first documented evidence is around the 11th century when the leaves and roots were used to cure many ailments. Many traditional dandelion cures have been passed down through generations, and the dandelion is well implemented as a useful product. The dandelion is a prolific grower as any gardener will tell you, but does not seem to grow as well in the southern hemisphere.

The young green leaves are extremely nutritious, the roots are an exceptionally good substitute for coffee and the flowers can be made into jam. The lowly dandelion stands as a regal plant amongst herbs and healing medicines.

Growing dandelion greens

Choosing dandelions ~ If you live in the northern hemisphere, it is unlikely that you will have to make a choice at all. The dandelions best grown in your area will undoubtedly come up all on their own. Let them seed and you will have a bountiful crop for many years. However, they are considered a weed by many gardeners and are stubborn to remove from the vegetable patch once they get a hold, so if you can contain the seed, it would be better for your garden as a whole.

When the seed head turns into a white, fluffy head full of seeds, sprinkle them over a prepared site and they will grow there; the seed is light and easily carried by the wind so a non-windy place would be best. Dandelion seed isn't readily available to buy, although a specialist grower could perhaps supply enough to get you going. The best way to obtain your dandelion seed is to collect it yourself. Look out for the seed heads in fields or woodland in early to late summer, or offer to weed your neighbour's vegetable patch and keep the dandelions!

Prepare the site ~ If you are preparing a specific site for your dandelions, dig over the patch and remove any weeds and large stones. Rake over to a fine tilth. The ground should be well-drained. Dandelions are very hardy plants and will usually be able to extract the nutrients they need from the soil with their long taproots, no matter what the condition of the soil. However, if you want to produce a good crop, a little feeding wouldn't go amiss. Dig in some well-rotted manure or compost early in the year before sowing the seed.

Position ~ Normally a sunny position is best for most yellow flowering plants, but dandelions have been known to grow inside dark sheds. A bright airy patch is best, but not necessarily in full sun. Dandelions often come up of their own accord in the middle of your lawn or the vegetable patch. If you can, leave them to mature and clip off the flower just before the plant starts producing seed. If you leave them to seed, it's highly likely you'll have a dandelion lawn next year.

Sowing dandelions ~ Once you have bought or collected your seed, and prepared your site, scatter the seed over the fertile earth and the dandelions will grow. Otherwise, just leave them to come up where they choose.

Caring for dandelions ~ Apart from cutting them down with the lawnmower I can't honestly imagine how you could fail at growing dandelions. They are one of the hardiest plants on the planet. In times of extreme drought they may suffer, but even then they are likely to survive longer than other plants because of their long taproot.

Poly-tunnels and Containers
There doesn't seem to be much point as dandelions are such a prolific and hardy plant. Even if you live in a flat or apartment and don't have access to a garden, dandelions grow just about everywhere. However, don't pick them from the side of the road as they will have absorbed some pollution.

Storing
Dandelion root can be stored for several weeks if kept in a dark place away from damp and mice. The flowers are best made into a preserve and stored in jars. The green leaves are best eaten fresh.

Raspberries

History
Raspberries are thought to have been available in many parts of the world in prehistoric times, although the first recorded use of cultivated raspberries wasn't until the 16th century. And it was as late as the 18th century when particular types and strains were listed.

Although they haven't been cultivated for many centuries, raspberries have always been a popular fruit and considered to be helpful in recuperating from illness as well as forming part of a healthy afternoon tea.

Growing raspberries
Choosing raspberries ~ There are a number of different varieties of raspberry including golden fruiting types. These are very attractive and taste just as good as the red raspberries. Browse soft fruit catalogues to find the variety you prefer and order it direct, or try your local garden centre. Raspberries tend to be adaptable plants and will grow in many climates, so don't necessarily stick to varieties that are grown locally.

Buy healthy canes with good root structure or, as with blackcurrants, a few canes cut from another grower's raspberry bush will develop roots within a year or two.

Raspberries are said to be one of the easiest fruits to produce, even for a novice gardener, so experiment a little. You may be pleasantly surprised.

Prepare the site ~ The soil should be well-drained and acid if possible. In the summer months, dig in well-rotted manure or compost.

Position ~ Raspberries, as most fruit, like a sunny location, but I've found raspberries growing prolifically behind garden sheds, although they don't produce quite as much fruit in shady spots, so choose a sunny part of the garden if you can. They make good border plants and can help to form a useful hedge. Use canes or trellises to help support the plants and you can create a very practical and nourishing hedgerow.

Planting raspberries ~ Raspberries are best planted in autumn or early winter but can be planted at the end of winter before the spring growth starts, if necessary. The first year may not develop as many fruits though if planted as late as early spring.

Place some stakes on one side of your intended row, and fix a strong wire between them at about 2-1/2 ft. (75 cm.) high, then a couple more spaced evenly up to about 5 ft. (almost a metre). Dig a trench along the row and place your raspberry canes about 12–18 in. (30–45 cm.) apart along the row. Leave about 2–3 ft. (60–90 cm.) between rows. Fill the trench and firm each plant in with your heel. Using a sharp pair of secateurs (pruning shears) cut each cane down to about 10–12 in. (25–30 cm.) straight after planting.

Caring for raspberries ~ In the following spring, the raspberries may have sent up new suckers, which can be removed and re-planted in a new row. Every year these suckers should be removed to help the main plant produce a healthy crop of raspberries.

At this time, mulch with a good, organic material. Raspberries are heavy feeders and should be fed fairly regularly with an organic fertiliser.

By the summer new canes should be growing and the original cane can be cut down to ground level. Tie the new canes to support wires. These new branches will produce fruit. Later on in the summer, when the canes have finished fruiting and you have collected the raspberries, the canes that produced fruit can be cut down.

Raspberries fruit on new wood so keeping the old wood cleared keeps the row tidy and the crop healthy and abundant.

Poly-tunnels and Containers

Check on the variety you buy for indoor growing recommendations. Most raspberries are hardy and don't require the extra heat and protection of greenhouses and poly-tunnels.

Raspberries aren't really adapted to container growing as they need a fair amount of space for root growth and they also grow quite tall, requiring stakes and wires to support them later on.

Storing

Fresh raspberries will only keep for a day or two but they can be frozen or bottled. Fruits can be bottled in alcohol to preserve them, but the fruit will absorb some of the alcohol so isn't suitable for children or anyone who prefers not to get intoxicated while eating dessert!

Freezing quickly will work but the texture changes dramatically when thawed. The best way to freeze raspberries is to make a pie or tart and freeze the whole dish in a suitable container. Remember to label. The dish will keep for a few months in the freezer. Another way to store raspberries successfully is to make jam or jelly. See Chapter Fifteen for recipes.

Sunflower Seeds

History

Sunflowers are believed to have been grown for thousands of years and probably originated in America. Through the 16th century, sunflowers spread across Europe and in the 18th century Russia put great importance on the cultivation of huge sunflowers. One of the types we buy today is called 'The Russian Giant' These plants can grow more than two metres tall and develop hundreds of oil producing seeds.

Because the sunflower seed is so rich in oils and minerals, it has become a commercial goldmine! We snack on seeds, cook with sunflower oil and the oil has even been used to replace diesel in controlled testing environments. The sunflower has an extensive root system and has been used to extract toxins from water supplies. On top of all that, it looks great in your garden or inside in a floral arrangement.

To grow sunflowers for the oil is usually not practical for the average gardener. Many thousands of seeds are required and the process of producing oil is time consuming unless the correct machinery and tools are used. However, you can grow enough sunflowers in your garden to produce seeds for snacks for the family.

Growing sunflower seeds

Choosing sunflowers ~ There are many different varieties of sunflowers and if you live in a particularly windy area, and have no wind breaks available, a shorter variety is probably easier to grow. However, the very tall types are stunning and are really worth growing if you can. Children love them!

You can find sunflowers in different colours but if you are growing them for seed, you should check whether the seed is edible. The huge, yellow sunflower is a glorious sight in the garden and you could leave a few of the plants for the birds and squirrels. Grow a couple of flowers just outside the kitchen window so you can watch the birds through the autumn.

Prepare the site ~ If you can, dig in some well-rotted manure or garden compost before sowing. The flowers will benefit from the extra minerals in the soil. Dig over and remove all perennial weeds. Rake to create a fairly fine tilth to plant your seed. The ground should be well-drained.

Position ~ The sunflower likes a sunny position and if possible, not too windy. Remember they grow very tall and the flower heads are large so they may shade other plants that are close by. Sowing next to a fence or even the wall of the house can work well. You could even stake them if you feel it's necessary. Make sure you put the stakes in before sowing though or you could damage the roots.

Sowing sunflowers ~ Sunflowers don't like to be re-planted so it's best to plant them where they will grow. The seed should be planted fairly thinly around 2 cm. deep. Place a line of stakes next to the seeds. Make sure the stakes are firm and won't blow over in a wind. When the seedlings come up, the plants should be thinned to allow around 50 cm. all round for each plant to develop. If you plant the seed sparingly you won't waste as many. Water the area well and keep watered and weeded until your plants become established. As the plants grow taller, secure to the stakes gently with a natural garden twine.

In general, sunflowers are easy to grow and make a great children's gardening project. They grow quickly and in the right weather conditions you can almost watch them grow in front of you!

In colder climates, you could start your seeds in bio-degradable pots and plant out later. Planting the whole pot into the ground saves disturbing the roots and the sunflower will carry on growing none the wiser. You should get them used to being outside though. Put them out for a few hours every day during the middle of the day if you can, and bring them in again at night until the weather is warm enough to plant them out permanently.

Caring for sunflowers ~ Sunflowers need very little looking after once they become established. Watch for wind damage and tie to the stake every now and then. If you intend to grow the seeds for yourself and your family, you'll need to protect them from birds and in some areas squirrels as well. Squirrels can chew through the stem and stroll off with the whole seed head in its mouth before you get up in the morning; I've seen them do it!

Once the flower has died back and the seed head starts to droop, you can remove it from the plant and dry it indoors. Cut the stem allowing around 30 cm. to use to tie up. Hang in a dry place, not in direct light, and tie a paper bag around the seed head to catch the seeds as they dry and fall out. Puncture a few holes in the bag to allow air circulation and keep the mice away.

Sunflower seeds are so popular with so many different species of wildlife that it can be a real battle of wits to end up with any yourself. However, if you don't fail to save them from the birds, squirrels or mice, at least you've done your bit for the environment and had the pleasure of beautiful sunflowers in your garden all through the summer months.

Poly-tunnels and Containers

There's no reason why sunflowers shouldn't be grown indoors, as long as they have enough light and height. Perhaps a few in a poly-tunnel would be a good idea to save them from the squirrels and mice. Make sure the ground is well-drained as they won't survive if their roots are in waterlogged soil. But keep watered at all times and weed free in the earlier weeks of growth.

Storing
When you've collected the seeds, spread on a baking sheet and sprinkle with salt and a little oil (both optional). Bake in a moderate oven for around 30–40 minutes. Leave to cool and store in airtight jars.

Chapter Ten

Growing Plants Rich in Folate

Beetroot, Green Beans, Parsley, Turnip Greens

Beetroot

History
It seems that the round, red beetroot we enjoy today didn't appear until the 17th century. Before that time it is thought to have originated from a sea plant that grew over many parts of the Asiatic and European coastlines. Beetroots were grown for their leaves at that time and the root was fairly insignificant.

However, the roots were used in medicinal preparations and since Roman times, beetroot has been used to treat various ailments and conditions, including fevers and constipation. The juice from beetroot was also believed to be an aphrodisiac. It does contain a mineral which plays a part in producing sex hormones so this is probably a well-founded belief.

The beetroot has been proved to contain so much natural sugar, vitamins and minerals in the root that it is a valuable crop for both humans and animals. It is grown extensively across the globe and is a very practical and nutritious vegetable.

Growing beetroot
Choosing beetroot ~ There are a number of different varieties available. Browse through a seed catalogue or two before heading down to the garden centre. Some varieties will produce a larger root than others, while some will be grown specifically for their leafy tops and will have very thin roots.

The root of the plant is by far the superior part, and there are many different sizes and shapes to choose from. Choose baby beets if you are growing in containers or pots. Experiment and grow a couple of different varieties every year.

Prepare the site ~ Beetroot doesn't like a very acid soil so add a little lime before sowing if necessary. Dig over during the autumn before next year's sowing season. Don't add manure as this causes the roots to fork. Remove any non-organic debris, perennial weeds and large stones.

Position ~ A light and airy situation is best for root crops, not necessarily in full sun. They won't thrive in shady positions but partial shade won't do them any harm.

Sowing beetroot ~ Sow in late spring after threat of frost has passed.

Beetroot seeds are 'multiple' seeds so don't need to be sown thickly. Sow thinly along the line, one seed cluster every 2–3 in. (5–7 cm.) and water after sowing. Allow about 12 in. (30 cm.) between rows. Don't start off in pots if you want to grow them later in the vegetable garden. As with most root crops they don't like to be moved and will not develop properly if transplanted.

You can start a few beetroots off earlier in the year by covering with a cloche and removing later on when the weather improves. Place the cloche over the soil for a week or two to warm it up before sowing the seed.

Caring for beetroot ~ The seedlings are fairly quick to germinate and should be up in about 2 weeks. Watch out for birds at this stage. It may be necessary to net the beetroot until they have grown a little bigger. Birds will peck a little at the leaves when the beets have grown but won't be able to pull them out of the ground.

Keep weeded and watered all through the growing season. If using a hoe, be careful not to damage the roots. Hand weeding is better if possible.

Thin to allow 4–6 in. (10–15 cm.) of growing room in each line. Double check on your seed packet as some varieties will need more space than others. It's okay to pick a few early leaves although care should be taken not to damage the growing stem.

Early roots are always worth treating the family with. They are very sweet when young and quick to cook. Don't leave them in the ground too long, and definitely not as late as the first frosts of winter. They should be lifted when the roots are not much bigger than 3 in. (6 cm.) in diameter, after that they tend to get woody and less sweet. The foliage starts to wilt when they have finished growing. Lift carefully with a trowel, not a fork, and ease the roots gently from the soil. Be extra careful not to damage the roots. Twist the tops off or cut the leaves an inch or two above the root to avoid 'bleeding'.

A few beetroot plants can be left to go to seed and the seed collected to plant the following season. However, beetroot will not seed until the second year, so will need a little extra looking after. Occasionally a plant will go to seed in the first year; whilst these seeds are usable they are often not as viable as seed produced in the second year.

Poly-tunnels and Containers

Beetroot can be planted a little earlier in a poly-tunnel or greenhouse, but they may run to seed quickly if too warm and dry. Check on your seed packets, as some varieties will be more resistant to bolting than others. Starting off beetroot under a cloche or a temporary poly-tunnel is a good way of getting a few early beets.

Baby beets are perfect for container growing. The container should be fairly deep, well-drained and not allowed to dry out.

Storing

The most traditional way of storing beetroot is by pickling in vinegar. It is possible to simply add cooked beetroot to vinegar in an airtight jar. The natural sugars in beetroot help conserve them.

Beetroots can be stored for a number of weeks in a dark dry place. Twist the tops off when lifting and don't store any damaged roots. Use any less than perfect beetroot immediately

Green Beans

History

Green beans, also known as bush beans and string beans, have been cultivated since the 16th century but a stringless variety wasn't developed until around the turn of the 20th century. Most green beans grown today will be stringless if picked at the right time.

Green beans are eaten as a whole pod before the bean inside develops. Beans can be left on the plant to develop the bean inside the pod, but these beans will probably have to be dried and stored for winter months rather than eaten green.

Growing green beans

Choosing green beans ~ There really are hundreds of different varieties of green beans. Buy a high cropping variety that is adapted to your region. Some are very long and thin and are suitable for different recipes. The average French type bean, or bush bean is very well suited to everyday eating.

Climbing beans, also eaten as a whole pod before the beans inside develop, are a good garden vegetable to grow. They can be grown along the border or up a tepee type structure to save space in the vegetable garden.

Beans are low in calories and high in vitamins and minerals. They should always be cooked before eating as they contain a poisonous substance in their raw state.

Prepare the site ~ Dig over the ground and clean out any non-organic debris, large stones and perennial weeds. Green beans are quite adaptable to most soil types.

Climbing beans need support and can be grown along a line of chicken or pig wire supported by stakes. Or a tepee structure can be made using long poles tied together. Stake each pole firmly in the ground and tie the tops together with strong string. Using a natural twine, run lines around the poles, wrapping round each one to secure. Leave about 8 in. (20 cm.) between each line.

Position ~ Green beans like a sunny spot in the vegetable garden. Short bush varieties grow well in border positions.

Sowing green beans ~ After all danger of a frost has passed, beans can be planted. Plant a short line every two or three weeks right through the spring and summer months to ensure a fresh supply. Green beans need to be picked as soon as they are ready to eat and not left too long on the plant. If left they start to develop the bean inside the pod and the pod becomes woody and inedible.

Beans grow and produce fruits very quickly and don't need to be started off earlier in a greenhouse or indoors. From around May, depending on how late you have a frost in your region, plant individual beans every 2–3 in. (5–6 cm.) along the row and cover with soil. Water well. For climbing beans, plant around the outside of the tepee as close as possible to the poles, or close to the netting for border growing positions.

Don't be tempted to soak beans before sowing. They can become easily damaged and fail to germinate.

Caring for green beans ~ Keep watered and weed-free. Green beans have a fairly delicate root structure and hoeing should be done very carefully if at all. Hand weeding is best.

If the weather is dry, spray the flowers with water when they start to form, twice a day or as often as possible. This helps set the flowers and ensures the beans get a good start.

Always pick beans before the bean inside the pod starts to develop. Leave a few on the plant if you want to store dried beans for the winter. The younger they are picked the more tender and sweet they are.

Poly-tunnels and Containers

Green beans will grow in poly-tunnels and greenhouses but make sure they get plenty of water, especially when the flowers start appearing.

Beans will also grow in containers, but tend to be happiest growing in lines fairly close together, in the open air and space the vegetable garden affords.

Storing

Green beans will store for a number of days after picking. Pick in the evening or early morning to avoid the midday sun making them floppy.

They can be frozen fairly successfully. Top and tail, take off any bits of branch and leaves and bag them up in suitable freeing bags. Label and freeze quickly. They will store for many months in the freezer.

Green beans can also be blanched before freezing. Immerse in boiling water for 4 minutes. Cool quickly, either in ice or cold, running water. Bag and freeze immediately.

Green beans can also be bottled or canned.

Any large beans not picked can be dried in airtight jars and stored for winter use.

Parsley

History

Parsley has been cultivated since at least 300BC and has been treated as a wonder herb as well as the 'devil's' herb over the centuries. The Ancient Greeks used to adorn graves with parsley and the Romans garnished every meal table with it. During the early years, parsley was mainly used as a healing herb and was believed to absorb bad odours and protect against intoxication from wine. In medieval times parsley was believed to bring bad luck. This myth probably derived from the importance the Ancient Greeks placed on adorning graves with the herb. Thankfully the myth was dropped and parsley has become one of the most used herbs in the western world.

Growing parsley

Choosing parsley ~ There are a couple of common parsley types. The most common, curly-leaved variety is used as a garnish for many meals or the flat-leaved, Italian variety that is favoured more by chefs for its stronger taste. Both can be used in cooking and as garnish. There are always new hybrid types of herbs and vegetables appearing in our garden centres and for the sake of a small increase in the budget, it's worth experimenting

Prepare the site ~ Parsley prefers a rich soil; it's best to dig in as much well-rotted manure or compost as you can before sowing. Remove large stones, stubborn weeds and any non-organic debris from the soil.

Position ~ Parsley likes to grow in full sun. It can be grown in rows in the vegetable patch or you can scatter it around the garden. It's nice to have a plant or two close to the kitchen door or even in pots on the windowsill. If the herb is right in front of you, it's easier to use it.

Sowing parsley ~ Start the seeds off indoors about two months before planting out. Planting out should be after all threat of frost has passed. Check on your seed packets for variations and regional recommendations. Sow a few seeds in each pot and keep them watered and warm. When the seedlings come up, leave the strongest looking one in the pot and discard the rest. You can try re-planting these weaker plants but it's probably better to add them to the salad bowl. A few strong plants will provide all the parsley you can use.

Parsley can take a long time to germinate. Make sure the pots are well-drained and the soil is kept moist during this period and you will be rewarded with strong, healthy plants.

Parsley seed can be sown directly outside but it does need a fairly long growing season. In moderate and cooler climates the plant doesn't have time to mature before the winter sets in. When the weather is warmer and the soil is warm and workable you can move the plants outside. Re-pot into larger containers if necessary or plant directly into the ground.

Give the plants at least 12 in. (30 cm.) of growing space all around. Follow the directions on your seed packets. For larger growing varieties you may have to allow a little more space.

Caring for parsley ~ Once the long taproot of the parsley plant has taken hold you shouldn't need to worry about it too much. Give the plants a little organic feed once a month to keep them producing more leaf. Parsley does need plenty of water though. If the roots dry out, the plant will suffer dramatically. Keep weed-free.

Cut stalks for use regularly, from the outside of the plant. Cutting stalks will encourage the plant to produce more foliage. Leave a couple of inches of stalk when you cut. You can start cutting when stems have reached at least 20 cm. in height.

Parsley is a biennial and in most climates, the plant will over-winter so you should be able to pick fresh parsley on even the coldest of winter days. Remember to add it to stews and soups. The vitamins and minerals will help prevent colds and flu.

The plant often runs to seed very early the following year, making it unusable. However, you can collect the seed and save for re-planting. Or use the root to add to soups and stews. Plant parsley every year so you have a good, healthy crop at all times.

Poly-tunnels and Containers

Parsley can be grown successfully indoors. Grow in pots or any well-drained container. Keep the plants in the lightest part of the house, usually on a windowsill. Conservatories are great places to grow your herbs but they mustn't be allowed to dry out. Set up a watering system if you're going to be away for a few days or more.

Parsley will also grow well in greenhouses and poly-tunnels but again, make sure the soil is kept moist and weed free.

Storing

With a little careful planning you should be able to produce fresh parsley most of the year, but for those other times it can be stored:

Drying: Simply hang whole stems or lay them on racks, turning regularly, in a cool, dry and airy place. When completely dry, crumble leaves and store in airtight, glass jars. Remember to label the jars.

Freezing: Parsley will freeze quite well. Freeze whole stalks quickly and store in sealable freezer bags or plastic containers. Label and date.

Turnip Greens

History

Turnips have been cultivated for at least 4000 years; the root was a food crop for man and animals for many centuries. Turnips were once considered to be a very valuable crop. They were used in trading, to cure illnesses – including measles – and even turned into an alcoholic drink.

Turnips were a very popular vegetable until potatoes became more available. But lately, many gardeners are growing a variety that doesn't produce such a defined root, but has plenty of foliage. These turnip greens are becoming more and more popular with the home gardener.

Growing turnip greens

Choosing turnip greens ~ To grow turnips simply for the greens, get one of the hybrid varieties available. However, turnip greens can still be eaten from the tops of regular turnip roots as long as the main stem isn't damaged. The greens are higher in vitamin and mineral content than the roots. Growing the root crop as well provides a double harvest for your family. Turnips are as nutritious as any other root vegetable.

Prepare the site ~ During the season before sowing, dig over the ground. Remove any large stones or non-organic debris. Work the ground fairly deeply for all root crops. For varieties of turnip grown just for the greens, the ground doesn't need to be worked so deeply. The land should be well-drained but not dry. Turnips mustn't dry out during the growing season.

Position ~ Turnips like an open, airy site but not full sun. Partial shade will work well.

Sowing turnips ~ Turnips are a cool season crop and will become bitter and even woody during hot dry periods. In hotter climates, they are best grown during the winter months, and in some moderate climates, avoiding very warm summers is preferable.

Plant seed thinly in lines about 12 in. (30 cm.) apart. Water when needed. Plant seed very early in the spring for summer harvesting and in late summer or early autumn for winter crops. The later turnips will tolerate a light frost or two, and the roots often become slightly sweeter after the first frost.

Turnips grown for the greens only won't need this frost to sweeten the root, and care should be taken as the new hybrid varieties will have different needs. Check on the seed packet.

Caring for turnip greens ~ When the seedlings are a few inches (5–7 cm.) tall, thin to around 4–6 in. apart (10–15 cm.). Put these thinned out seedlings in the salad bowl, a soup or stew. These tiny plants are very rich in vitamins and shouldn't be discarded.

Pick a few roots when they are fairly small. Young vegetables are always more tender and often higher in vitamin and mineral content. Pick the leaves gently, taking care not to damage the centre growing points, and the plant will keep on producing leaves right through the season. Use them while they're young and tender. All leafy vegetables tend to be more bitter as they get older.

Keep well watered and weed free. The turnip root has few enemies and should just get on with growing until ready to harvest.

Poly-tunnels and Containers

Containers aren't particularly suitable for growing root crops. It may be possible, but the container will have to be fairly deep, well-drained and the soil kept moist at all times. However, the varieties grown specifically for greens could be grown in pots and would be useful to keep a few around the house. Young turnip greens can be used in salads.

Turnips won't benefit from indoor growing, so greenhouses and poly-tunnels aren't really a suitable environment. They are a cool climate crop, so there isn't any point in using up valuable inside space for turnips. It would be necessary to keep them cool and other plants that need the warmth would suffer.

Storing
Most leafy greens don't store very well as they are. Make a soup or other dish with your turnip greens and freeze quickly in suitable containers. Remember to label. Turnip roots will keep for a couple of weeks if stored in a dark, dry place.

Chapter Eleven

Growing Plants Rich in Niacin

Aubergine (Eggplant), Courgettes (Zucchini), Fennel, Peas

 Aubergine

History

Aubergines, or eggplants, have been around for over 2000 years and probably originated in Asia. It wasn't until the 16th century that they were brought to the west and another century passed before aubergines were accepted as edible vegetables. For many years they were grown as ornamental plants.

Aubergines have had bad press over the centuries. They belong to the nightshade family and were thought to be a dangerous fruit to eat. Immature plants do carry some toxins akin to the deadly nightshade plant. But the mature fruits are perfectly safe to eat and with hybrid varieties available, there is no risk to health unless you have an actual allergy to them.

WARNING: do not eat the small immature fruits.

They are a warm climate plant but can be grown successfully in most parts of the world. In cooler climates, a cloche or greenhouse may be advisable to protect the plants from extreme weather conditions.

Growing aubergine

Choosing aubergine ~ There are different varieties from which to choose, such as: yellow and white aubergines as well as the very attractive and more familiar, purple types. Purple vegetables are more likely to have a richer vitamin and mineral content. There are also different shapes: some are longer and slimmer than the regular pear shape, some are very round and come in varying sizes.

Many aubergine plants grow fairly large and bushy and will need a fair amount of space to fully develop. If the space is available, try a couple of different varieties.

Prepare the site ~ Aubergine likes a rich, and preferably sandy, soil. Add well-rotted compost during early spring before planting out. The ground should be moist but never waterlogged.

Most varieties need support. Place stakes in the ground firmly before planting.

In cooler climates, including northern Britain, aubergines will need to be grown in poly-tunnels, greenhouses or under cloches.

Position ~ Aubergines are a warm weather vegetable and prefer being in direct sun, although with the new, hybrid types it would be advisable to double check on growing recommendations on the seed packet. They will not tolerate frosts or even very cold nights and cloches or greenhouse growing may be advisable depending on your climate.

Sowing aubergine ~ In a moderate to cool climate, seed will have to be started off inside; a greenhouse, conservatory or bright, sunny room in the house will do. Plant seed in a tray or pot of seed compost and keep moist and warm. Too little light will make the plants straggly and weaken them. Keep in a bright spot and not too hot but never let them get cold. Sometimes getting the balance right can be tricky. Read growing recommendations on the seed packets and stick to them carefully.

If sowing outside, make sure all threat of frost has passed and the nights are warmer. In cooler climates plant out under cloches, in a greenhouse or poly-tunnel. Allow about 2–3 ft. (60–90 cm.) of space all round each plant and water.

Caring for aubergine ~ Keep aubergines free of weeds, especially during the early weeks. When the plants are around 18 in. (45 cm.) tall, pinch out the top of the main stem to encourage more side shoots. Side shoots should carry no more than one fruit each although some smaller fruiting varieties may support more. Check which variety you have and read the growing recommendations.

They are heavy feeders and should be fed regularly with an organic fertiliser but only a little each time. Little and often is best for aubergines. The same applies to watering. They need watering very regularly, especially in dry conditions, but mustn't be over watered. In heavy rainfall areas, it's best to protect the plants.

Cloches should be available to quickly cover your aubergine patch. They are a fiddly crop to grow in anything but a tropical climate where they will thrive with very little attention. But they are worth the effort and once the system has been perfected, as with everything, they will be a rewarding plant to have in the garden.

Poly-tunnels and Containers
Aubergines are happy in poly-tunnels or greenhouses, especially in cooler climates. They are a warm weather crop and don't appreciate cold nights or chilly days.

Aubergines are suitable for container growing but some plants can become quite bushy and the container will have to be fairly big and well positioned to grow well developed fruits. Place a stake in each pot before sowing to avoid damaging the roots. Aubergines will grow in pots in a conservatory or a bright, sunny windowsill.

Storing
Aubergines will keep for a few days in the salad compartment of a refrigerator. They can be stored in a freezer but will keep better if made up into a dish, such as ratatouille, beforehand. Put into a suitable container, label and freeze quickly.

Courgettes

History

Courgettes, or zucchini, are part of the large squash family. Most squashes originated in America but courgettes appear to be native to the Mediterranean area of Europe. The Italians probably started eating immature marrows and from that point on they became a vegetable in their own right. Courgettes didn't become popular in Europe or America until the early 20th century.

Growing courgettes

Choosing courgettes ~ There are so many different squashes that it can be very confusing to try and group them into any sort of order. The courgette is part of the same group as pumpkin and apart from the pumpkin leaves being a lot larger, the two plants are very difficult to tell apart before the fruiting stage.

Choosing courgettes can be equally as confusing as there are a number of different shapes, sizes and even colours to choose from. The regular, green, cucumber-like courgette is the most popular, and if left to grow large will become a marrow. There are yellow varieties and also round shaped courgettes. I have grown round courgettes very successfully for many years and they are just as delicious as the long shape, although it's preferable to eat them when young and small. One healthy courgette plant will produce many fruits. A couple of plants from a few different varieties will provide interesting shapes and colours for the dinner table.

Prepare the site ~ Soil must be well-drained but moist. Dig in well-rotted manure or compost in the autumn or early spring. Many growers like to grow squash plants on a mound, and courgettes have been known to come up of their own accord in compost heaps.

Position ~ Courgettes like a sunny spot in the garden, but can tolerate a partially shaded area. Check on the variety you are sowing, as some types will be more tolerant of shade than others.

Sowing courgettes ~ Start early courgettes in a greenhouse or other warm place. Sow 2 seeds in small pots, and discard the weaker plant later. Biodegradable pots are preferable to avoid damaging roots when transplanting. But courgettes are fairly hardy plants and will tolerate being removed from pots and transplanted outside quite comfortably.

Keep the soil in the pots moist at all times. Squashes are high in water content and need plenty of water to grow well. They shouldn't be left in waterlogged soil though, so make sure the pots are well-drained. Protect against slugs and snails.

Keep warm for a few weeks until the plants have 3 or 4 true leaves (not counting the first two). Choose a warm day, when all threat of frost has passed and the soil has warmed up a little.

Before planting out soak the pot then ease out gently. Try to avoid touching the roots. Plant out in the morning and allow about 2–3 ft. (60–90 cm.) of space all around for them to grow. When they are small, this seems like a huge area, but they will very quickly grow into the space they're allowed. Courgettes are one of the fastest growing plants and always surprise even the most seasoned gardener with their rapidity of growth.

Water well and protect against slugs and snails. Use an organic product or try using crushed eggshells placed carefully around each plant. Don't leave any gaps in the circle or the slugs and snails will surely find the way in.

Another way is to place a circle of plastic with salt or other dry, sharp medium, such as sand, around the plants. Or you could try a long board on either side of the row with sand and sharp gravel poured on it. If you have problems with slugs and snails, and most gardens do eventually, try anything to deter them. Frogs and toads keep the population down and are worth encouraging into your vegetable patch.

Courgette fruits tend to come thick and fast when they start producing and it's a good idea to plant a few plants in the early part of the year and then plant seed directly outside in the middle of summer. The plants will grow quickly and will provide a late summer, early autumn crop.

Caring for courgettes ~ Once the plants are in position outside, and the slugs haven't devoured them, courgettes will get on with growing all by themselves. However, they do need watering and won't thrive if allowed to dry out.

Keep weed free during the early weeks. When the plants are bigger the abundant foliage will shade the ground and it's unlikely they will allow any weeds to get in their way.

Cut courgettes as they become available. Use a sharp knife and cut just above the stem. Pulling the fruits will damage the plants. Use the first courgettes when they are small. The plant will be encouraged to grow more and before you know where you are, you won't be able to keep up with them. Courgettes are said to be one of the easiest vegetables to grow in the home garden, even for the beginner.

If you get fed up with courgettes and your plants are still flowering, try eating the flowers. Dip them in batter and cook for a few minutes in hot oil. A delicacy worth trying!

When the plants have finished producing, they will easily pull up and compost very quickly.

Courgette seeds are also a nutritious food and can be collected from mature fruits, dried and eaten raw or roasted. Store in airtight jars when totally dried. Hamsters and mice love them!

Poly-tunnels and Containers

Courgettes can be grown in containers but they will need to be fairly large to accommodate the fruits as they grow.

They can be grown in poly-tunnels, greenhouses and under cloches. In a very cool climate they will do well under glass or plastic. In most moderate climates though, once started off, they will grow happily outside.

Storing

Courgettes will keep for a week or two in a cool, dark place. If left to grow into a large marrow they will keep for a few weeks providing there is little humidity.

Courgettes can be sliced, laid out on suitable trays and frozen quickly. Store in containers and label. The courgettes won't keep their crisp texture though, as with most vegetables, once frozen they become softer and less appealing, and they also lose some of their vitamin content.

Courgettes can be pickled very successfully and many mustard pickles have courgettes in the recipe. Pickle just courgettes and maybe a little cauliflower for an acceptable everyday preserve.

Fennel

History

Fennel has been cultivated for thousands of years and was used as a healing herb as well as a food crop. The Romans believed it helped eyesight, while the ancient Greeks believed it helped weight problems. Fennel has quite a reputation for being a slimming aid. The Anglo Saxons considered it to be a sacred herb. The leaves and seeds were used in healing and flavouring foods and the bulbous root became popular during the Middle Ages. At one time, fennel was used in almost every meal as it aids digestion, contains no fat at all, and is a good source of vitamins and minerals. The strong anise flavour and odour helps to repel insects.

Growing fennel

Choosing fennel ~ There are a few varieties of fennel, some will be specifically grown for the bulbous root, and others can be grown for the leaves and seed. With a little careful cultivation, both can be achieved from the same plants.

Prepare the site ~ Fennel grows very tall and will need support in windy weather. Place a few stakes where you intend to plant your seed. Position the stakes well and press firmly into the ground.

Fennel will grow in most types of soil but prefers a richer soil if possible. Choose a well-drained area and don't grow fennel in waterlogged sites.

Position ~ Fennel shouldn't be planted near dill or coriander and it can also affect a tomato crop. Fennel is a sun worshipper and a full sun position is most suitable.

Fennel plants can grow as tall as 6 ft. (2 m.) so they need to be positioned where they won't throw too much shade on other plants. Lettuce can be grown fairly close as they prefer a little shade.

Choose a non windy spot if possible.

Sowing fennel ~ As soon as the soil is workable (late spring or earlier if possible), fennel seed can be planted. Fennel doesn't like to be transplanted but if you need to start the plants earlier in the year, they can be started in biodegradable pots to avoid damaging roots and tricking the plants into thinking they haven't been transplanted at all.

Sow seed thinly in lines about 18–24 in. (45–60 cm.) apart. Sow as close as possible to the stakes or support system already in place. Water gently. When the seedlings are a few inches (5 cm.+) high, thin to allow around 12 in. per plant. Water each plant carefully.

Caring for fennel ~ Keep weed free and watered especially during very dry weather. Fennel prefers a rich soil and will benefit from a couple of organic feeds during the growing season.

Fennel will naturally die back during the cold weather and doesn't need any attention.

It will also seed itself, so by leaving one or two plants to do their own thing, you will undoubtedly get lots of baby fennel plants popping up in the spring. They can be invasive if you have fairly mild winters. The seed will tolerate a number of frosts, but may not survive a prolonged freeze.

To fully develop the bulbous root, the soil should be drawn up around the base of the plant after the plant is fully grown and left to swell and blanch. When the bulbs are large enough to use, pull up alternate plants in the row, and let the others grow on. Check on the seed packets for your particular variety as each type will have different needs.

Poly-tunnels and Containers
Fennel can be successfully grown in poly-tunnels and greenhouses, and will very likely produce larger bulbs than if planted outside. Again, be careful of the seed dropping and regrowing the following year as the plant can overtake an area very quickly

Containers work as well, but the fennel plant does grow tall and will need a fairly deep container to mature successfully.

Storing
Fennel bulb will keep for 4 or 5 days in a refrigerator. Or make a soup or other favourite dish, pour into a suitable container, label and freeze quickly. It will keep for many months.

Fennel seed is worth collecting, and kept in an airtight jar will keep well for months. Fennel leaf can be frozen or dried. To freeze, lay on suitable trays and freeze quickly. Bag and label. To dry, hang in a dark place and crumble into an airtight jar when completely dry.

Peas

History
Peas have been cultivated for human consumption for thousands of years, but it wasn't until the late 17th century that the pea became a popular vegetable to eat fresh. Before that time it was used as a dried crop. Dried peas were taken on long sea journeys as they were light to carry and highly nutritious for the crew and passengers. Peas can be stored almost indefinitely. They are a cool

weather crop so don't require long, hot summers to thrive. In fact the regular pea plant is better planted early in the season and harvested before the weather gets too hot.

As soon as the pea became a popular fresh vegetable, cross breeding started taking place; we now enjoy many different varieties of peas, including the shelling type with a very fibrous pod, and sugar peas which have virtually no 'pea' inside but can be eaten whole and are very sweet. These peas are often used in stir-frys and salads.

Growing peas

Choosing peas ~ There are many different types of pea you can grow in the home garden and within each type there are many varieties. The regular garden pea has a fibrous shell and the peas inside should be removed from the pod and eaten raw or cooked until soft. I have many childhood memories of shelling peas with my grandmother and eating as many as I could before they reached the saucepan. Try it with your kids!

Another 'pod' pea is the marrowfat type which is left to grow until quite large and used in dishes such as 'mushy peas' and stews as a warming winter vegetable.

'Mange tout' or 'sugar snap' peas can be eaten whole. They are best eaten just before the tiny peas inside start to develop. After that the pod gets fibrous and not good to eat. The whole pod is particularly sweet and nutritious, can be eaten raw or cooked and is a great favourite with the children.

There are many other varieties of peas that can be grown in the vegetable garden. Have a look at the varieties available in your garden centre. These will most likely be good to grow in your area. Ask experienced local gardeners as well. You could try yellow peas and other special types.

The other thing to decide when growing peas is the height the plants will grow to. Some are dwarf varieties and will grow into neat, little bushes, but others will need huge support systems. I use 'pea-sticks' for medium high plants. Pea sticks are random sticks or canes with small branches to support the peas. (The plants send out tendrils to wrap around their support system and it helps if the surface isn't too smooth; birch twigs or last year's raspberry canes are good for this.) For higher growing plants, use a roll of pig wire staked into the ground at intervals. Peas do very well with this kind of support system.

Prepare the site ~ The first crop of peas can be planted very early in the year so it's best to try and prepare your patch during the preceeding autumn. Dig over, remove any stubborn weeds and large stones etc; and cover with an organic mulch or simply old carpets or cardboard. Covering the soil like this prevents the soil from becoming too frozen if the winter gets harsh and also discourages early spring weeds.

If you haven't been able to prepare before winter, dig over gently as soon as you can and spread a little well-rotted manure or compost over the ground. Don't add nitrogen to your soil as peas 'catch' nitrogen from the air and store it in their root system. When the pea plants have finished cropping and die back, digging the withered plant into the soil sets nitrogen for your next crop of vegetables. Next season's peas should be planted in another part of your garden as the soil in this year's area will probably be too high in nitrogen content for them. Peas will grow in nitrogen rich soil but will be very leafy and won't produce a lot of fruits.

Peas should be grown in the same patch as beans and preferably not with other vegetables in your garden. Peas and beans are legumes and do like to have a place of their own.

Remember to place the supporting pea sticks, wire or netting when you've prepared the ground before you start sowing your peas.

Position ~ Generally, peas are a cool climate crop and they grow very well in the UK and cooler parts of the United States. They don't need direct sun but will thrive in a bright and airy spot. Try and organise a patch especially for your peas and beans as they grow well together. I often grow peas around the edge of the vegetable patch next to paths and walkways. This makes it easier to pick the peas as soon as they are ready. Although peas and beans grow well together and make perfect companion plants, beans need slightly warmer weather and should be planted later than peas.

Sowing peas ~ Make sure the ground isn't waterlogged. Peas do need a well-drained soil. Plant peas 3–5 cm. deep and 5 cm. apart in rows. Rows should be at least 40–50 cm. apart. You need to reach the peas and therefore enough space should be allowed to walk between rows and hoe gently when necessary.

Some growers advise soaking the peas in water for a few hours or overnight to speed up the germination process. I have also heard of gardeners soaking the seed in paraffin to deter mice and birds. And yes they are a problem. I've had whole rows of peas disappear in a couple of hours.

Some form of covering that lets light through can be used to protect your seeds until they start sprouting. They tend to germinate quickly considering the size of the seed. You will probably find a whole row of tiny pea plants within 10–14 days. Always double check the instructions on your seed packets as different varieties will require different growing conditions.

Caring for peas ~ With favourable conditions, you can almost watch peas grow! They send out very strong tendrils which they use to grip the support sticks and these supports should be in place before you sow the seed.

Peas don't need too much water and will not thrive in water logged soil. Don't mulch around the plants as the stalks will rot very quickly and the plant will die.

When the flowers have been out for a couple of days, you will notice a small pea fruit growing from the middle of the flower. Keep an eye on them at this stage. Within a couple of days these pea pods will be ready to eat if you wish. Mange tout varieties can be eaten as small as you like and definitely shouldn't be allowed to get big enough to be growing small peas inside the pod. If you do miss a few, these peas can be used in a stew rather than a stir-fry. Check for stringiness.

Poly-tunnels and Containers

Peas tend to like cooler climates and indoor growing may not always be good. However, there are many hybrid types on the market now and you may find a particular variety especially made for greenhouse or conservatory growing.

Containers would work in theory but most peas need some sort of support to climb up, so unless you grow a particularly short growing variety, containers aren't very practical.

Storing

Peas can be frozen, bottled, canned or dried. They are probably the most versatile of all vegetables when it comes to storing.

Freezing: Young, fresh peas can be possed and spread out on plastic trays and frozen quickly. Pour into bags, label and put back into the freezer.

Bottling and canning: If you are set up for these processes, peas can be bottled or canned and kept almost indefinitely.

Drying: Peas can be dried in the sun if the climate is hot. Use a dryer or oven in humid conditions. Shell peas and blanch in steam or boiling water for a few minutes. Cool, then lay out on sheets ready for drying. Dry for 5–9 hours in a dryer if you have one. However, for home use an oven is usually large enough to dry your peas.

Set the oven to its lowest setting and keep the door open slightly when drying. Place trays of peas in the oven and 'heat' for a few hours, until totally dried. Turn the trays every half hour or so. Don't stop and restart this process as any moisture left in the peas can turn to mould and spoil the whole crop.

Chapter Twelve

Growing Plants Rich in Pantothenic Acid

Broccoli, Cauliflower, Chicory, Parsnip

roccoli

History
Although broccoli has its roots in ancient times, the broccoli plant as we know it today, wasn't cultivated until the 16th century in Italy. It probably started in Mediterranean areas and travelled through Asia before returning to Italy. The vegetable slowly made its way across Europe and America over the next few centuries. It wasn't commercially produced and didn't become an everyday vegetable until the 1900s. Now broccoli has a reputation of being a super-food and contains many healthy vitamins, minerals and antioxidants.

Growing broccoli
Choosing broccoli ~ There are a few different varieties of broccoli, including a purple sprouting variety which is attractive as well as being delicious and high in vitamin and mineral content. Try a couple of different types or check which are most suited to your region.

Prepare the site ~ Most brassicas don't like an acid soil, so lime should be added before sowing if necessary. Dig in plenty of well-rotted manure or compost during the season before planting out. Remove any perennial weeds, large stones and non-organic debris from the ground. Although broccoli is a fairly hardy plant it prefers a nice, clean soil if possible.

Do not grow brassicas in the same place two years running in case there is cabbage root fly in the soil.

Position ~ Broccoli likes full sun but will cope with partial shade. Some broccoli can stay in the ground during winter months, so it's best not to plant where there is likely to be a heavy frost pocket or the soil is likely to get water logged. Keep out of windy areas if possible.

Sowing broccoli ~ Different varieties of broccoli will have different sowing needs and it's best to check the sowing recommendations on your seed packet before you start.

Generally, to have broccoli ready to harvest in late summer and autumn, seed should be started in early spring. Seeds need a fairly warm germination period, and should be started off in a greenhouse or conservatory in mid-April or earlier depending on the climate in your region. Plant the seed in fairly rich compost in trays. Remember to label the tray, especially if you are growing other brassicas. They all look very similar at the seedling stage. Keep warm and watered until the plants have about 4 or 5 true leaves and the weather has warmed up.

Broccoli seed can be started off outside using a cloche. Place a cloche over the area for a couple of weeks to warm up the soil before sowing. Plant thinly and leave at least 2 ft. (60 cm.) between rows. Seed started outside should be sown a little later or when all danger of a frost has passed.

Caring for broccoli ~ Once your seedlings are ready to plant out, they should be watered well before removing from pots and care should be taken with handling. Try not to disturb the roots too much as this could cause damage to the growth of the plant.

Transplant into prepared ground allowing about 18–24 in. (45–60 cm.) between plants and at least 2 ft. (60 cm.) between rows. Again double check on the seed packet for spacing advice.

Keep your broccoli crop well watered, but never let it get waterlogged. And don't let the weeds take over.

When the heads are ready to eat, cut through the stem with a sharp knife and eat the same day to get the most benefit. Leave the plant in the ground as broccoli will usually send off lots of little branches and produce many more heads. These new shoots will produce smaller broccoli head than the main stem but they are still just as delicious.

Don't leave the heads until they flower as they become bitter. If you have more than you can use fresh, either give them away or freeze quickly.

Poly-tunnels and Containers

Broccoli will grow in containers as long as they have enough depth of soil and are not allowed to dry out. Always keep containers well-drained and well watered.

Some varieties may not do well in poly-tunnels or greenhouses. Check on the growing recommendations on your seed packet.

Storing

Broccoli will store in its fresh form for up to a week in a cool, dry place. It can be successfully frozen. Break into small florets and freeze quickly on trays. Put into suitable containers or bags and label. Broccoli will keep in the freezer for many months.

Broccoli can also be made up into a meal before freezing. Soups and stews freeze well and are useful to have in the freezer for busy days when there's no time to prepare a proper meal. Rather than resort to a fast food alternative, dip into a ready, home-made meal.

Cauliflower

History

Cauliflower originates from the cabbage plant which has been cultivated for thousands of years. It went through various transformations through the ages and became popular as the cauliflower we know today in the Mediterranean area during the 1st century. It wasn't until the 16th century that it became a popular vegetable across Europe and the 17th century before it was grown in America.

Cauliflower became available as a commercial crop in the UK early in the 17th century but didn't become a commercial crop in America until early in the 20th century. Cauliflower is almost the same plant as broccoli but is more tender and needs a little more care during growth.

Growing cauliflower

Choosing cauliflower ~ There are different types of cauliflower available, including seasonal varieties. Cauliflowers can be grown all year round given the right growing conditions. Check on the packet when you buy cauliflower seed to ensure you are getting the right variety for the time of year and your climate. Some summer varieties are harvested in summer but sown in winter under glass, but other summer varieties are sown outside in spring for late summer harvesting.

Prepare the site ~ Cauliflower should not be grown on the same ground where brassicas have grown during the previous 2 years. They are very susceptible to disease, more so than other brassicas.

Cauliflowers like a non-acid soil and are heavy feeders. Balance your soil with lime previous to sowing if the acidity levels are too high. Dig over the ground in the autumn for spring sowings, and incorporate plenty of well-rotted manure or compost. Add a layer of good organic fertiliser to the surface after digging. For winter sowing, cauliflowers are hardier and won't need so much fertiliser. Dig in the manure previously but don't add the layer of fertiliser to the surface area.

Position ~ Cauliflowers like full sun and will not develop properly if in the shade or near to trees. They are very particular about their growing space so should be given the best position in the vegetable patch if possible. Avoid windy spots. Winter sown varieties like to be sheltered from the worst of the winter weather.

Sowing cauliflower ~ There are many different varieties of cauliflower and each will have its own unique sowing schedule. Read the recommendations on the seed packet and stick to them.

Generally for late summer and autumn harvests, the seed will need to be started in the spring under glass. Start off your seed in trays of rich seed compost and keep warm and watered until the weather is warm enough to transplant into the vegetable patch.

For early spring harvest, seed will need to be started in late summer directly outside if the weather is warm. But winter cauliflower needs a lot of warmth to germinate so you may have to start the seed off under glass. Depending on the severity of the winter in your region, it's advisable to have a cloche available to protect the young plants as they start to develop. Winter grown cauliflowers grow more slowly though and some varieties will be fine during the winter months without protection.

Avoid windy spots or particular frost pockets.

Caring for cauliflower ~ Cauliflowers do need more attention than other brassicas but the end result is worth the extra work. When the soil has warmed up in the spring, the early sown varieties will need planting out. Summer grown cauliflowers grow quickly and need huge amounts of food to develop properly. Feed them regularly with an organic fertiliser and keep watered.

Make sure the ground is never waterlogged or dried out. The plants need to be in a moist, rich soil to fully mature. Summer growing cauliflowers need watering all the time and it may be a good idea to set up an irrigation system if you live in a region with hot, dry summers. As soon as they start to dry out, the heads will stop growing and won't mature well. Winter growing cauliflowers can have a problem with too much water. Grow on a ridge to help with drainage. There are very defined growing conditions needed for different types of cauliflower and it can be tricky getting the balance right. Following the seed manufacturer's instructions is the most reliable way of producing a good harvest.

Cauliflowers are ready to eat when the leaves aren't covering the white edible part. They should be harvested straight away or they discolour. If the outer leaves can be pulled over the 'curds' they can be left for a few extra days. Secure with a natural garden twine. Cut in the morning and remove plants from the ground. Cauliflowers won't produce anymore, unlike cabbages or broccoli. If there has been a frost in the night, cut the cauliflower when it has warmed up and isn't likely to be frozen.

Poly-tunnels and Containers

Cauliflowers can be grown in containers, but extra care is needed with watering.

Poly-tunnels and greenhouses are possible with some varieties. Check on the seed packet to make sure you know which type you are growing. Every type of cauliflower has slightly different needs and won't thrive unless they have the perfect growing conditions.

Storing

Fresh cauliflower will keep for a week or so if kept in a dark place. Cauliflower freezes well. Break into individual florets and freeze quickly. Store in the freezer in suitable containers. Remember to label. Cauliflower will keep for several months in the freezer.

Cauliflower is also added to pickles and is a common ingredient in mustard pickle. It can also be made into soups, stews, casseroles and curries and frozen as a complete meal. Label and freeze quickly.

hicory

History
Chicory has been grown for thousands of years for its food and medicinal value. The ancient Egyptians grew chicory for medicinal use and the Romans grew it for the salad leaves and believed it had strong medicinal qualities. Over the centuries it became less popular and was grown for animal feed until the 18th century when coffee became very expensive. Instead of having to increase the price of coffee, the French started producing chicory to add to the coffee beans. The roasted and ground chicory root became so popular that it was enjoyed in many countries and still is today.

Growing chicory
Choosing chicory ~ There are many different uses for the chicory plant. The leaves can be used as salad greens; the roots can be pulled and ground to make a coffee substitute or added to coffee for the taste. And the roots can be forced in a dark place to produce endive.

Look through the seeds in your local garden centre as there will be different varieties available.

Prepare the site ~ Whilst wild chicory is very common on wasteland and will grow between the cracks in the pavement if allowed to, to get the best out of your crop, it's probably wise to prepare the site. Dig over the ground and remove any large stones, perennial weeds and non-organic debris. Chicory likes a rich soil so add some well-rotted compost if necessary.

Position ~ Chicory likes to grow in full sun while producing foliage. Later, to force the roots to produce endive, you will need a dark and fairly warm room, and a forcing container

Sowing chicory ~ Wild chicory will grow in the strangest of places and doesn't ever seem to need any particular looking after, but to grow the cultivated varieties a little care should be given to this wonderful diverse plant.

After all danger of a frost has passed, chicory seed can be sown directly outside. Make sure the ground has been well prepared and hoe the top few inches to a fine tilth. Alternatively the seed can be started off earlier in the greenhouse or indoors. Keep the seedlings warm and watered, and plant out when the weather has warmed up. Allow about 18–24 in. (45–60 cm.) between rows.

If chicory is being grown only for the leaves, sow the seed fairly thickly and cut and use as required. For roots and endive growing, sow seed more thinly as they will need spacing later on.

Water well.

Caring for chicory ~ Keep weed free and well watered especially during dry periods. Chicory leaves can be used anytime and should be cut as required.

For root growth, thin the seedlings to allow about 8–10 in. (20–25 cm.) between each plant. Double check on the growing recommendations for your variety as each will vary.

After 3–4 months, the roots will be ready for harvesting. When they are 1–2 in. (3–5 cm.) in diameter, they can be dug up and immediately 'forced' or roasted and ground to make a coffee substitute.

To 'force' your chicory, you will need a forcing container; it needs to be kept in a dark place in around 60 degrees to produce the white endive. Fill a deep container with fine soil and place roots in the soil so that the top of the root comes about level with the surface of the soil. Add a few inches of sand and water. Keep soil moist and store box in a dark, warm place for a couple of weeks. The roots will produce another 'head' which you can harvest as soon as it looks edible.

Poly-tunnels and Containers
Chicory will grow in poly-tunnels and containers but double check on your growing instructions first. Make sure the plants don't dry out.

Storing
Chicory root can be roasted, ground and kept for many months in sealed jars, and can be used as a coffee substitute.

Endive can be kept for a few days in a cool place or in the salad compartment of the refrigerator. Or make a meal with your endives and freeze. Put into a suitable container, label and freeze quickly.

Parsnips

History
Parsnips have been around for thousands of years and it's believed they were very popular with the ancient Romans. For many hundreds of years parsnips were grown as a hardy root crop and were one of the most important root crops of the time. The potato took over in popularity somewhat but the parsnip is making a comeback.

They will grow wild over many parts of Europe if left to their own devices. Because of their sweet flavour, they have been used in sweet as well as savoury dishes. In medieval England parsnip was used in bread and given to babies to soothe them. Parsnips have also been used for many years, especially in rural areas, to make wine and beer.

Growing parsnips
Choosing parsnips ~ There are a number of different varieties, like the carrot that they are related to; there are shorter, wider types and longer, narrower types. If you have a shallow soil the shorter ones would be more advisable to grow.

Prepare the site ~ Don't dig manure into the ground. As with all root crops, manure or rich compost will cause the roots to fork. Dig over and loosen the soil. Remove any large stones and non-organic debris. Pull up any perennial weeds and make the ground as clean as you can.

Position ~ Parsnips are a long growing vegetable and will occupy their spot for a large part of the year. If you have the space available, they are a wonderful vegetable to grow for winter use and can be left in the ground until required. But if space is limited, you may feel that giving over a spot just for parsnips for nearly a whole year may not be viable. Parsnips like full sun.

Sowing parsnips ~ Plant parsnip seed in situ; they do not transplant well, like all root crops. Parsnip seed tends to be erratic and germination is often very slow. It can sometimes be up to a month before you'll see signs of any seedlings. As they are very temperamental, plant thickly, and in lines about 18–24 in. (45–60 cm.) apart. Keep the ground moist but don't be too zealous with watering. The seed is very light and can be washed away easily.

Caring for parsnips ~ As soon as the seedlings are a couple of inches (5 cm.) high, thin to allow about 4 in. (10 cm.) between plants. Double check this spacing on your seed packet. Keep weed free and watered especially during the summer months while they are developing.

Parsnips are much better after the first frost, and although they are perfectly edible before, the frost does add that touch of sweetness particular to the parsnip. Dig up carefully to avoid damaging the roots anytime you want. The leaves can also be eaten; use the smaller leaves in salads. They resemble celery, to which the parsnip is also related.

Poly-tunnels and Containers

Container planting isn't as popular with root vegetables. It is possible but the container must be very deep, especially for parsnips. They have a very long taproot and need a lot of depth to fully develop. The container should also be well-drained but never allowed to dry out. Parsnips get sweeter after the first frost and containers can sometimes protect plants from frost, which works well for some plants, but not for parsnips.

Storing

Parsnips will keep in the ground right through the winter, but in very cold winters the ground may be too frozen to dig them up. If you are expecting the cold, dig up parsnips and store in a barrel of sand or in boxes in a dark place, as you would with carrots. Keep the mice away.

Parsnips will keep well in the salad compartment of the refrigerator for a few days, or in a dark, airy space. They will also freeze fairly well. Scrub or peel if necessary and cut into thick slices. Spread on trays and freeze quickly. Put into a suitable container or bag and store in the freezer for up to a year. Parsnip can also be stored as a ready meal, such as a soup or casserole. Put into a container, label and freeze. Or try your hand at making parsnip wine. A glass or two will warm the bones on a cold winter's night!

Chapter Thirteen

Minerals

Minerals are required for a healthy, fit body and are present in fresh food. Processed foods are often lacking in something, and minerals and vitamins can be dramatically reduced from fresh food in processing. By eating as much fresh food as possible, there is more chance of absorbing the vitamins and minerals we require every day. In addition, processed foods often have a higher refined sugar and sodium content.

There are processed foods with added vitamins and minerals and. within reason, these can be incorporated into a healthy daily diet. Take note of sugar, salt and fat content though.

The major minerals we require are:

- calcium
- potassium
- sodium
- magnesium
- phosphorus

And the trace minerals:

- iron
- iodine
- selenium
- copper
- zinc

Calcium

Calcium is an important mineral especially for bone health. 99% of calcium in the body is stored in our bones and an adequate supply is needed daily. It's also important for healthy teeth and gums. The daily recommended intake of calcium for an average adult between 19 and 50 is 700mg. The best source of calcium is dairy products.

Rich alternatives include:

- kidney beans – 27 mg. per 100 g.
- black beans – 28 mg. per 100 g.
- brazil nuts – 160 mg. per 100 g.

Good sources of calcium in garden vegetables per 100 g.:

Source	Unit	Raw	Cooked (no salt)
turnip greens	mg.	190	33
broccoli	mg.	47	40
kale	mg.	135	72

Phosphorus

Phosphorus is required by almost every cell in the body and 85% is stored in the bones. It's rare to have a phosphorus deficiency but it can happen when an individual has specific health problems. Phosphorus helps keep cells, bones and teeth healthy. The daily recommended intake of phosphorus for an average adult between 19 and 50 is 550 mg. The best sources of phosphorus are normally high protein foods such as dairy produce, fish and meat.

Rich alternatives include:

- brazil nuts – 725 mg. per 100 g.
- lentils – 180 mg. per 100 g.
- home produced baked beans – 109 mg. per 100 g.

Good sources of phosphorus in garden vegetables per 100 g.:

Source	Unit	Dry roasted (no salt)	Dried
sunflower seeds	mg.	1155	705
pumpkin seeds	mg.	1172	1174

Source	Unit	Cooked	Raw
baked potato with skin	mg.	70	N/A
mushrooms	mg.	105	86
broad beans	mg.	125	421
globe artichokes	mg.	86	90

Magnesium

Magnesium plays a role in energy and metabolism and can be reduced by alcohol abuse and ailments including renal failure. It is also important in controlling calcium in the blood and processing fat. The daily recommended intake of magnesium for an average adult between 19 and 50 is 300 mg. for a man and 270 mg. for a woman The best sources of magnesium are in wheat germ, dairy products and chocolate.

Rich alternatives include:

- brazil nuts – 376 mg. per 100 g.
- tofu – 60 mg. per 100 g.
- raw cashews – 292 mg. per 100 g.
- almonds – 275 mg. per 100 g.
- English walnuts – 158 mg. Per 100 g.

Good sources of magnesium in garden vegetables per 100 g.:

Source	Unit	Cooked (no salt)
spinach	mg.	87
broad beans	mg.	43

Source	Unit	Dried
green beans	mg.	18
broccoli	mg.	21
sunflower seeds	mg.	354
pumpkin seeds	mg.	535

Sodium

Sodium keeps the water balance in our bodies under control. High levels of sodium can lead to osteoporosis. In addition to keeping water levels correct, sodium plays a part in nerve impulses and muscle contractions. It also helps keep the acid/alkaline levels balanced. The daily recommended intake of sodium for an average adult between 19 and 50 is 1600mg. The best source of sodium is salt. Most processed or commercially prepared food is high in sodium. High levels of salt are not good and preparing your own food with a little salt is generally enough.

Other sources include:

- cheese, cheddar – 621 mg. per 100 g.
- olives, canned – 872 mg. per 100 g.
- packaged cereals etc; (check on packet)

There is only a trace of sodium in fresh garden vegetables. If no processed foods are taken on a daily basis it is enough to add just a little salt in cooking. Normally though this is unnecessary, as there is usually salt added to cereals, cheese, and other processed foods, however 'healthy' they may seem.

Potassium

Potassium, along with sodium, helps keep the acid/alkaline balance in the body. It also helps store sugar and is essential for muscle function. Recent studies have shown that potassium helps lower blood pressure and is therefore an important mineral for those with heart problems. The daily recommended intake of potassium for an average adult between 19 and 50 is 3500 mg. The best sources of potassium are whole grains, dairy products and red meat.

Rich alternatives include:

- brazil nuts – 659 g. per 100 g.
- avocados – 485 mg. per 100 g.
- bananas – 358 mg. per 100 g.
- oranges – 181 mg. per 100 g.
- melon – honeydew – 228mg. per 100g.
- melon – cantaloupe – 267mg. per 100g.

Good sources of potassium in garden vegetables per 100 g.:

Source	Unit	Cooked (no salt)	Raw
asparagus	mg.	224	202
spinach	mg.	285	558
tomatoes	mg.	218	237
broad beans	mg.	268	332

Source	Unit	Baked + skin	Mashed (home made)
potatoes	mg.	544	298

Iron

Iron is perhaps the most well known vitamin and lack of it results in anaemia – one of the most common nutritional disorders in the world. Iron builds and repairs the body and adequate iron should be taken everyday. Never overdose on iron though, as it can be fatal. The daily recommended intake of iron for an average adult between 19 and 50 is 8.7 mg. for a man and 14.8 mg. for a woman The best sources of iron are in meat, offal and fish.

Rich alternatives include:

- dried fruit – (prune, apricot and pear mixed) – 2.71 mg. per 100 g.
- chickpeas – 2.89 mg. per 100 g.
- raw Cashews – 6.68 mg. per 100 g.
- English walnuts – 2.91 mg. per 100 g.

Good sources of iron in garden vegetables per 100 g.:

Source	Unit	Cooked	Raw
spinach	mg.	0.80	2.71
broad beans	mg.	1.50	1.55
beetroot	mg.	0.79	0.80
green beans	mg.	0.65	1.04
parsley	mg.	No data	6.20

Source	Unit	Dried	Roasted no salt
sunflower seeds	mg.	6.77	3.80

Zinc

Zinc plays a great role in growth and development and is important to pregnant women and to sperm production in men. The daily recommended intake of zinc for an average adult between 19 and 50 is 9.5 mg. for a man and 7 mg. for a woman. Zinc is found in beef, chicken, oysters, shrimp and yoghurt.

Rich alternatives include:

- Brazil nuts – 4.06 mg. per 100 g.
- almonds – 3.36 mg. per 100 g.
- lentils – 1.27 mg. per 100 g.
- raw cashew nuts – 5.78 mg. per 100 g.

Good sources of zinc in garden vegetables per 100 g.:

Source	Unit	Cooked	Raw
mushrooms	mg.	0.48	0.45
potatoes (baked)	mg.	0.35	No data
peas	mg.	0.37	0.27
green beans	mg.	0.25	0.24
sweet corn	mg.	0.48	0.45
Source	Unit	Dried	Dry roasted
pumpkin seeds	mg.	7.46	10.30
sunflower seeds	mg.	5.06	5.29

Copper

Copper plays a role in energy metabolism, helps repair scar tissue and transports electrons around the body. It also plays a part in the function of the nervous system, and in processing iron. The daily recommended intake of copper for an average adult between 19 and 50 is 1.2 mg. Good sources of copper are found in offal, chicken, seafood, milk and chocolate.

Rich alternatives include:

- raw cashew nuts – 2.195 mg. per 100 g.
- Brazil nuts – 1.743 mg. per 100 g.
- almonds – 1.110 mg. per 100 g.
- dried prunes, uncooked – 0.281 mg. per 100 g.
- pistachios, dry roasted, no salt – 1.325 mg. per 100 g.
- sesame seeds, whole dried – 4.082 mg. per 100 g.

Good sources of copper in garden vegetables per 100 g.:

Source	Unit	Cooked	Raw
mushrooms	mg.	0.291	0.318
globe artichoke	mg.	0.233	0.231
turnip greens	mg.	0.002	0.350
Source	Unit	Dried	Roasted no salt
pumpkin seeds	mg.	1.387	0.690
sunflower seeds	mg.	1.752	1.830

Selenium

Selenium is a component in the chemical process that reduces free radicals. Deficiency is rare and supplements shouldn't be taken unless medically advised. Too much selenium can produce side effects such as nausea, irritability, loss of hair and brittle nails. The daily recommended intake of selenium for an average adult between 19 and 50 is 75 mcg. for a man and 60 mcg. for a woman. Selenium is found in offal, poultry, seafood, eggs and yoghurt.

Rich alternatives include:

- Brazil nuts – a staggering 1917.0 mcg. per 100 g.
- oatmeal, cooked with water – 8.1 mcg. per 100 g.
- brown rice – 9.8 mcg. per 100 g.
- tofu, fried – 28.5 mcg. per 100 g.
- raw cashew nuts – 19.9 mcg. per 100 g.

Good sources of selenium in garden vegetables per 100 g.:

Source	Unit	Cooked	Raw
mushrooms	mcg.	13.9	9.3
broad beans	mcg.	2.6	0.8

Source	Unit	Dried	Roasted no salt
sunflower seeds	mcg.	59.5	79.3
pumpkin seeds	mcg.	5.6	5.6

Iodine

Iodine is used solely in thyroid function and is a common deficiency in those with thyroid problems. The daily recommended intake of iodine for an average adult between 19 and 50 is 140 mcg. Iodine is not present in many foods and fruit and vegetables are dependent on the content of iodine in the soil for the iodine to be present in the plant. It is very unlikely, with a normal diet and a clean water supply, there would be any iodine deficiency.

Generally iodine is present in drinking water but can also be found in:

- seafood
- cheese
- eggs
- bread

There are other trace elements we require on a daily basis, although most are only needed in very small quantities and are easily available in a normal healthy diet. Sticking to healthy foods, and as far as possible, unprocessed, will generally provide all the minerals we require to stay healthy.

Chapter Fourteen

Herbs

Herbs have been used in culinary, cosmetic and medicinal preparations for thousands of years. There is scientific evidence of various herbs being buried with humans around 60,000 years ago. At that time they were probably thought to have supernatural powers. Over the millennia, herbs have become more accepted as natural plants with super healing powers, as well as being good to eat and useful for a number of other everyday needs.

Humans have always used herbs to flavour food, and fresh herbs will add a touch of elegance to any meal, whether it be an everyday family supper or an exclusive dinner party.

Grow a selection of herbs around the garden or in pots around the house so they are ready to pick. Herbs love to be used and will thrive if regularly cut and used.

Herbs to make you feel good

There are dozens, if not hundreds of garden herbs you can grow to add to recipes and treat minor ailments.

Herbs should never be taken in large doses as the strong medicinal properties can be overwhelming for the nervous or digestive system. A wine glass or two per day is plenty.

If you are taking any medication, check with your medical practitioner before treating yourself with herbal medicines. Herbs could cause a reaction, perhaps making the prescribed drugs ineffective.

Here are a dozen herbs that grow easily in a moderate climate and can be infused to make tisans for all the family (sweeten with a little honey if preferred).

basil	chamomile	nettle
blackberry / bramble	fennel	sage
blackcurrant	lemon Balm	thyme
borage	mint	yarrow

Basil

As well as enhancing every tomato dish you could think of, basil leaves are considered to have a calming and soothing effect. Basil has mild sedative properties and is helpful in treating stomach cramps and headaches.

Basil originates in Asia and grows wild in Mediterranean areas. It is a warm weather herb and an annual, so needs to be planted every year and kept warm.

Growing ~ Start seed inside in late spring and early summer. Plant in pots of rich organic seed compost. Keep soil moist. Basil doesn't like to have wet leaves or stems. Water from the base or pour water on surface of soil avoiding the stem.

Plant in full sun – a couple of plants around the tomato patch works well. Or in a more moderate climate, plant in containers and move the containers to follow the sun. Move inside or into a greenhouse or poly-tunnel if the temperature gets a little low.

Pick leaves as soon as the plants have a couple of branches and look strong enough. Keep picking as often as you like.

Later on in the year, basil can be carefully lifted from an outside growing position and planted in a pot to bring inside. Try not to damage the roots when lifting.

Basil can be dried and stored in sealed glass jars for winter use.

Blackberry/bramble

Blackberry fruits are delicious eaten straight from the plant, in pies and cakes and compliment apples beautifully in an apple and blackberry crumble. The fruits and leaves contain antioxidants that are instrumental in controlling free radicals and therefore helping heart disease and some cancers.

Blackberry or bramble leaf tea is a well known and used remedy for diarrhoea, sore throats and mouth ulcers. Because of its high vitamin and mineral content, it also acts as a good tonic.

Growing ~ Brambles tend to grow by the side of the road, along hedgerows and just about any piece of fertile land if allowed to. The brambles by the side of the road could absorb toxins from car fumes and shouldn't be picked. Also some hedgerows along farmer's fields that look rich and are dripping in blackberries aren't always as healthy as they look. There are farmers who still use chemicals on their land. These chemicals blow on to the hedgerow in the wind, or are taken up by the roots.

Stick to your own home grown plants and have a ready supply of wonderful fruits and medicinal leaves through a large part of the year.

Take a cutting or dig up a stray rooted plant from another gardener or buy a new plant from the garden centre.

Brambles are just about the hardiest fruit you could grow and will thrive in cooler climates quite happily. They need very little attention, but keep watered and weed free until established, and check on growing recommendations if buying a new plant.

Blackcurrants

Blackcurrants are another plant originating in cooler climates. Native to Northern Europe, the blackcurrant has quickly spread over the world as an important medicinal herb.

The currants are used extensively in drinks and food flavourings, and are famous for their healing powers. Blackcurrants are a good soothing herb for sore throats, coughs and colds. The leaves of the plant are said to have cleansing properties and will help rid the body of any stray germs and infections that may be present.

Growing ~ Blackcurrants must be pruned regularly to keep the plants healthy. For more growing details see blackcurrants in Chapter Eight.

Borage

Borage was said to be the herb of courage and was given to soldiers before battle.

Throughout history, borage has been credited with powers to drive away sadness and bring happiness to the soul.

It has been used externally to reduce inflammations, and as a tisan to help cure respiratory problems. Borage is also said to reduce fever and help stimulate milk production in new mothers.

Growing ~ Borage is a hardy plant and can become invasive in the garden if not checked. Many growers prefer to grow herbs in containers for this reason. Borage likes a very sunny position and prefers a rich soil. Dig in plenty of good organic compost before planting if you can.

Plant seed early in the year in small biodegradable pots and keep soil moist. Plant out when the soil and air temperature outside have warmed up, or replant in containers. Water well after transplanting.

Keep soil moist, especially if grown in containers. The ground should be kept well-drained and weed free.

Borage produces hundreds of star like blue flowers and will attract bees by the dozen, so if you're allergic to bee stings, don't keep the pot next to an entrance to the house.

Cut leaves as you need them. They can be added to salads (they have a mild cucumber taste) or drunk as a tisan to make you feel good any time.

Chamomile

Chamomile is one of the most well known herbs and is readily available in tea form in many supermarkets. Chamomile was worshipped by the ancient Egyptians because of its healing qualities, and was regularly used in medicinal preparations by the Greeks and Romans. It has traditionally been used as a remedy for nightmares.

Chamomile has successfully been used to treat such conditions as arthritis, stomach disorders including ulcers, and anxiety. The immune system is said to benefit from chamomile, and it is worth trying a tisan or two if a cold or flu is on the way. Chamomile has been used externally to prevent infection in wounds. It has also been used in shampoos and will lighten hair.

Flowers are used in teas and all preparations.

Growing ~ Chamomile seed can be planted after all danger of frost has passed. The seeds are tiny and should be scattered over a prepared site in the garden. The plants will not be happy in full sun, so choose a partially shaded site. Chamomile is often grown next to pathways and invades the path itself. Stepping on the herb allows its scent to fill the air.

In the garden, care should be taken, as chamomile is self-seeding and will become invasive if not checked. After scattering the seed, tamp down with the back of a rake or other suitable tool, and water gently. Very small seedlings can be transplanted but not larger plants. Keep ground moist and weeded until the herb becomes established.

Flowers are normally produced within a couple of months and can be picked and used as required. Leave a few on a plant to self-seed but be careful not to leave too many.

Fennel

Fennel has been used as a healing herb for at least 2000 years. It has mainly been used as a digestive aid and still is today. A fennel sauce with any meal will aid digestion and ease flatulence. Fennel has been reputed to help milk flow in nursing mothers probably due to the mild oestrogenic effect acting like the female sex hormone.

Fennel has been used in weight loss programmes but it is in fact a diuretic, and basically just removes water from the body. Fennel isn't advisable to take as a diet product. Healthy food and exercise is the only positive way to shed those pounds.

Bruise the seeds with a wooden spoon and add to boiling water. The taste is similar to liquorice. Use the leaf in tisans, as well as sauces and salads.

Growing ~ Fennel shouldn't be planted near tomatoes or green beans. And coriander growing nearby will affect its development. For more growing instructions see Fennel in Chapter Eleven.

Lemon Balm

Lemon balm, originally from Europe but now grown all over the world, was used as a medicinal herb in Roman times and possibly before. During the Middle Ages lemon balm was thought to have youth restoring powers and was collected and sold across Europe. Lemon balm soothes and calms, and has been one of the most important herbs of the last 2000 years. It has mild sedative properties, and can help anxiety disorders. It will also aid digestion, and ease irritation from insect bites. A leaf rubbed on a recent mosquito bite will reduce the itching significantly. Lemon Balm is a wonderful herb to alleviate cold and flu symptoms, and refreshes the whole body.

Herbs with sedative properties can lower the effectiveness of thyroid medications, and also should not be taken by pregnant women or nursing mothers.

Growing ~ Lemon balm isn't fussy about the soil it is grown in, but will thrive best in fertile soil. Lemon balm prefers a fairly shady spot and will develop more quickly there than if planted in full sun. Lemon balm can grow very tall and can be invasive so choose your spot well.

The seed is very small and is better started in seed trays in a warm environment. Cover with a very light layer of seed compost and keep the compost moist until the seedlings appear. As soon as the seedlings are big enough, plant out in the garden and water well. Keep watered and weed free and the plant will look after itself.

Cutting from the plant can be started as soon as it's established. Cutting will encourage more growth.

Mint

Mint is another ancient healing herb and has been used to soothe pain throughout history. It is commonly used these days to aid digestion, hence the need to eat after dinner mints. A cup of mint tea will probably serve the body more successfully than a chocolate mint though.

There are many different varieties of mint, the most common being spearmint and peppermint, and all types can be added to many meals, including salads. Chop a couple of leaves into a salad bowl for an extra zing. Add mint leaves to new potatoes, fresh peas, and make a fresh mint sauce to serve with lamb dishes.

Mint tea will help digestion and has been found to aid irritable bowel syndrome, stomach cramps, flatulence and many other ailments. A cup every day will soothe digestion problems, and may clear tension headaches without resorting to tablets.

Growing ~ Another invasive herb if not checked. Many growers prefer to grow mint in pots to avoid it taking over the whole herb bed. If grown in pots extra care needs to be taken with watering. It will die if left unattended, however hardy it may be.

Start seed or cuttings in early spring and keep watered and weed free until established. Once it is well rooted it will choke out any weeds that attempt to grow. Cut and use mint as often as you can. It will keep producing as quickly as you can use it. If you want to store mint for the winter months, cut down to almost ground level just before flowering. If you're not sure when this is, look out carefully for the first flower to appear, then cut immediately. Hang upside down in a dark cool place until dried and crumble into glass jars. Keep lid on to keep flavour in.

Nettles

Nettles are probably the most invasive plant you can have in the garden, so if you choose to have a nettle patch, keep well away from children's play areas and keep under control. Nettles are worth having around. They have healing properties and are rich in vitamin C. The young leaves can be cooked and eaten like spinach. Cooking eliminates the sting.

Nettles are used in cloth manufacture and have been since the Bronze Age. The leaf has been found to reduce blood sugar levels and high blood pressure. (Note: if you are taking prescribed medication for any of these conditions, check with your medical practitioner before treating yourself with nettles.)

Nettles are believed to be good for boosting iron supplies in the blood, and are also considered by many to be a cleanser and therefore excellent as part of a detox diet.

Nettles have been said to cure eczema and even arthritis.

Growing ~ Nettles can be grown from seed, but are probably easier to get going by digging up an unwanted root from a neighbour's garden. Ask first though! They will grow in more or less any conditions and must be carefully controlled or they will invade the whole garden. Cut down when flowering to avoid seed spreading. Use young leaves as they grow. Always use protective gloves when dealing with nettles.

Sage

Sage is probably best known for the wonderful smell it produces when cooked with a Christmas turkey or Sunday roast. As well as its great culinary powers, sage has important medicinal uses. Throughout history, sage has been considered to be an herb that can cure just about anything from cuts and bruises to mortality. Sage isn't a cure-all, but does have many important healing properties that are used in herbal preparations around the world today. It helps reduce sweating and has been administered to menopausal women to reduce hot flushes. It is a natural antiseptic and anti-inflammatory plant that can be used externally to treat wounds.

It is also said to be effective in treating anxiety disorders and depression, and is a useful tonic and stimulant. A glass of sage tea a day will certainly blow the cobwebs away and make you feel good.

Growing ~ Sage seed should be started indoors in early spring in trays of organic seed compost. Plant small seedlings out when all danger of frost has passed. Sage likes a well-drained soil and a full sun position. It likes a fertile soil but is quite a hardy plant once it gets going. In very cold winters it is wise to cover with a mulch to protect the roots from freezing.

Keep watered and weed free during its first year of growth until established. It doesn't mature for two years and shouldn't be used during the first year. For immediate sage availability, take a cutting from another plant, or buy a sage plant from a garden centre.

Sage likes to be kept moist but won't tolerate waterlogged ground. It's very susceptible to mildew. Sage will grow into a fairly large bush and will go on for years, however, it does tend to get woody when mature and it's advisable to renew plants every 3–4 years.

Thyme

Thyme has been used as a healing herb for many centuries; it was used by the Romans to treat various complaints. Thyme is considered to be a calming herb for those suffering with nervous disorders or depression. A pillow of thyme is a much used remedy.

Thyme is a very useful culinary herb and is added to a variety of meals, sauces and salads. The leaves and flowers can be infused to soothe coughs and colds. Thyme leaves are useful as a quick first aid application for minor wounds as it is a strong antiseptic.

Thyme tea can help stomach cramps and menstrual pain but should not be taken by pregnant women as it can relax the uterus. However, a small amount of thyme in cooking is safe.

Growing ~ Thyme can be started from seeds, cuttings or even root division. The growing area should be well-drained and in full sun.

Start seeds off indoors as they need a warm environment to germinate. Plant seed in a tray or pot of seeding compost. Keep warm and watered but do not let the soil become waterlogged. Plant out when all danger of frost has passed allowing around 12 in. (30 cm.) of space all round for growth.

To start your plant with a cutting, cut a stem from an established plant and push cut end into moist sand. The stem should produce roots in a couple of weeks. Plant out when weather is warmer. Water.

For root division, dig up plant very carefully, keeping as much soil on the roots as possible. Gently pull apart into two or three clumps and replant in moist soil at least 12 in. (30 cm.) apart.

Thyme prefers a drier soil than most plants and should never be over-watered. Make sure the soil is well-drained. Thyme plants do well on top of stone walls or next to paths. Keep free of weeds until plant becomes established

Yarrow

Yarrow has always been used to treat wounds – as far back as Roman times soldiers were told to rub the crushed plant on flesh wounds. The plant has chemicals that are antiseptic, anti-inflammatory, pain relieving and even help to congeal the blood, making it a very effective herb to treat flesh wounds.

Yarrow also helps aid digestion and smoothes muscular tension in the digestive tract. It has been used to treat a number of medical conditions over the years. It is claimed to regulate menstruation and also ease tooth pain. Since science has proved a lot of these claims to be possible, yarrow turns out to be a very worthwhile herb to grow in the home garden.

Yarrow has mild sedative qualities so shouldn't be taken in large doses, especially not before operating machinery or driving. A cup of yarrow tea, made with the leaves and flowers before bedtime is the perfect end to the day.

Growing ~ Yarrow seed can be started in spring under glass. Plant in seed trays or pots of fairly rich organic compost and keep warm and moist until the seedlings are big enough to plant out and all danger of frost has passed. Seed will take a couple of weeks to germinate. Plant out seedlings in a full sun position in well-drained soil. The soil mustn't be water logged but yarrow needs watering regularly to develop well. A little organic plant food is advisable if your soil is very poor in nutrients but normally yarrow will thrive in most soil types, as long as it's well-drained.

Yarrow can be propagated by root division. Dig up carefully and replant. This should be done every few years to give the plants space to grow. They will produce more foliage and flowers if allowed some space.

Use fresh leaves and flowers in tea. Use leaves and flowers as a quick first aid garden plant for small cuts and grazes.

To store yarrow, it should be cut and hung upside down in a cool dry place until completely dry. Keep stems in a sealed container to retain goodness.

Try as many different herbs as your space allows. Many herbs can be grown in containers around the house. Herbs can be enjoyed around the garden.

Chapter Fifteen

Recipes

The following recipes include conversions for all measurements.

Asparagus

Fresh asparagus is ready to cut during the 'hungry gap' in the vegetable garden – before the early summer lettuces and other vegetables get going – and lends itself well to warming dishes. Don't let the asparagus rot in the ground, cut it and eat it!

ASPARAGUS – THE ROYAL VEG

Asparagus is a wonderful vegetable to serve as an accompaniment to almost any meal. Steam or boil lightly. Drain well and toss in a little butter. Experiment by tossing a few mixed herbs into the pan after draining or even a crushed clove of garlic. Serve with a wedge of lemon or lime.

ASPARAGUS SALAD

ingredients
asparagus spears
chopped nuts
walnut oil / any other preferred dressing

method
~ cut raw asparagus spears into short lengths and mix gently in a bowl with chopped nuts
~ stir in oil or salad dressing
~ sprinkle a few chopped herbs over the top or stir into salad before adding dressing

If you prefer your asparagus cooked, steam gently for a few minutes, drain and cool before mixing with nuts.

ASPARAGUS OMELETTE

ingredients
asparagus spears (2–4 spears per omelette)
eggs (allow 2 per person for a main meal or 1 per person for a snack)
grated cheddar cheese or crumbled feta cheese
sunflower oil

method
~ steam asparagus gently for a few minutes until tender but not too soft and keep warm (allow 1–2 asparagus spears cut into very short lengths per person)
~ beat eggs well and stir in cheese
~ heat a little sunflower oil in a frying pan and pour egg mixture into pan

~ add cut asparagus and cook gently for a couple of minutes

~ turn omelette over and cook for a further few minutes until egg is set

~ fold omelette in half and serve with one or two uncut asparagus spears on top

~ serve hot with a green salad

ASPARAGUS SOUP

ingredients

1 lb., 450 g. or 3-1/2 cups asparagus

3 oz., 75 g. or 6 tbsp. butter or low-fat equivalent

1 or 2 medium sized onions

2 pts., 1 litre or 5 cups chicken or vegetable stock

seasoning to taste

method

~ cut asparagus and onions into thin slices

~ melt butter in a large pan and gently cook vegetables until starting to soften

~ add the stock and bring to the boil

~ turn down heat and simmer for about 40 minutes until the vegetables are tender

~ season with a little salt and pepper or a few mixed herbs if preferred

~ serve immediately

As an alternative, put through a blender and serve as a creamy soup.

For a touch of elegance, swirl a little single cream into soup just before serving.

Chill soup for a couple of hours and enjoy straight from the fridge.

Asparagus is a wonderful vegetable for soups. It can be cooked with potatoes, leeks or any mixed vegetable soup.

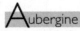

Aubergine

Aubergines are a good source of fibre and can be used in many dishes. To extract bitter juices: slice in half lengthwise and sprinkle cut surfaces with a little salt. Leave for 30 minutes and rinse. Then use as required.

STUFFED AUBERGINE

ingredients

2 aubergines

4 slices of chopped ham or 1 small can of drained, flaked tuna

finely chopped, mixed herbs to taste

1 can chopped tomatoes or 4 very ripe tomatoes chopped

6 oz., 50 g. or 1-1/2 cups grated hard cheese (such as parmesan)

method

~ preheat oven to 350F, 180C, or gas mark 4

~ cut aubergines in half lengthwise and remove bitter juices (see above)

~ place in a baking dish with a little water and bake in the oven for 45–50 minutes

~ carefully scoop out the flesh and mix in a bowl with ham or tuna, mixed herbs, and chopped tomatoes

~ spoon mixture back into aubergine cases and sprinkle cheese on top

~ grill under a moderate heat for 5–10 minutes

AUBERGINE PIE

ingredients

2-1/4 to 2-1/2 lb., 1 kg. or 4–5 cups aubergines
10 oz., 275 g. or 2-1/2 cups grated hard cheese
4–6 tbsp. grated parmesan
1–2 finely grated or crushed cloves of garlic
4 eggs
6 tbsp. fresh breadcrumbs (or mixture of chopped nuts and breadcrumbs)
finely chopped herbs to taste (e.g. oregano, basil, coriander)
salt and black pepper

method

~ preheat oven to 350F, 180C or gas mark 4
~ peel and cut aubergines into chunks
~ remove bitter juices (see above)
~ mash flesh in a large bowl and stir in the cheeses, half the breadcrumbs, garlic and herbs
~ beat the eggs lightly and add a little salt and plenty of black pepper
~ stir the egg mixture into the aubergines
~ spread mixture into a lightly greased baking dish and sprinkle breadcrumbs over the top
~ bake for 35–40 minutes

FRIED AUBERGINE

ingredients

aubergines
oil
batter mix:
    4 oz., 125 g. or 1 cup flour
    1 egg
    1/4 pt., 150 ml. or 1/2 cup milk or milk and water

method

~ slice aubergines and remove bitter juices (see above)
~ make batter:
~ place flour in a bowl and make a well in the centre
~ break in the egg and add a little of the milk
~ gradually fold the flour into the liquid and slowly add the rest of the liquid
~ beat well until smooth
~ dip each aubergine slice into the batter
~ fry in a little hot oil or deep fry for a few minutes until batter is golden brown

RATATOUILLE

ingredients

1 lb., 450 g. or 2 cups aubergines, sliced
1 lb., 450 g. or 3 cups courgettes, sliced
1 lb., 450 g. or 4 cups onions, chopped
1 lb., 450 g. or 2-1/2 cups tomatoes, chopped or 1 large can tomatoes
1–2 cloves garlic, crushed
chopped mixed herbs to taste
3 medium peppers (green, red, yellow or orange or a mixture)
olive oil

method

~ cut aubergines into thin slices and remove bitter juices (see above)

~ cut courgettes into fairly thin slices

~ cut onions into rings or chop finely

~ remove seeds and slice peppers into rings

~ chop tomatoes roughly

~ heat a little oil (olive oil is best but any light cooking oil will do) in a large pan

~ cook the garlic and onions gently for a few minutes, taking care not to burn

~ add the rest of the ingredients and stir well

~ cover and simmer for about an hour until all vegetables are tender

~ serve hot or cold

Beetroot

Beetroot has traditionally always been pickled to store as a nourishing vegetable for the winter months. But there is so much more that can be done with the humble beetroot.

Choose small to medium beetroots and twist off the tops to prevent the colour and goodness seeping out during cooking. Boil for around 30 minutes or until tender. To test, press on beetroot with your finger, careful you don't burn yourself. If the skin starts to peel away it's cooked.

Serve hot as it is or with a parsley sauce, or serve cold.

APPLE AND BEETROOT SALAD

ingredients

8 oz., 200 g. or 1 cup cooked beetroot, sliced

4–6 oz.,100–150 g. or 2 cups red lettuce leaves

2–3 red apples

2 oz., 50 g. or 1/4 to 1/2 cup almonds or walnuts

juice of 1 lemon

method

~ dice apples and toss in lemon juice to prevent discolouration

~ put apples into a large bowl or serving plate and add lettuce leaves

~ slice beetroot

~ add to salad and toss in a dressing of your choice

~ sprinkle nuts over the salad

Dressing suggestion:

    2 tbsp. olive oil

    1 tbsp. nut oil

    1 tbsp. cider or wine vinegar

    black pepper

    ~ mix all ingredients well

BEETROOT AND POTATO SALAD

ingredients

4 beetroot

4 potatoes

1/4 pint, 150 ml. or 1/4 to 1/2 cup natural yoghurt

1 red onion, finely chopped or grated

1 small green pepper finely chopped

parsley leaves to garnish

method
~ steam or boil beetroot until tender
~ drain and leave to cool
~ dice and peel (if desired) and dice potatoes
~ steam or boil until just cooked
~ drain and leave to cool
~ chop beetroot and mix in a bowl with potatoes and onion
~ in a small bowl, mix yoghurt with green pepper
~ stir most of the yoghurt mixture into the vegetables
~ spoon the rest of the yoghurt over the salad
~ add parsley leaves to garnish

BEETROOT SOUP

ingredients
6 small beetroots
2 stalks celery
1 onion
1 parsnip
1–2 carrots
1–2 cloves of garlic
2-1/2 pts., 1-1/4 litres or 6 to 6-1/4 cups of chicken or vegetable stock
a little cooking oil

method
~ chop onion and garlic
~ slice celery
~ place in a large pan with a little water and cooking oil
~ cook gently for about 4–5 minutes until soft
~ peel and grate beetroot, parsnip and carrot and add to pan with stock
~ bring to the boil and simmer for 30–40 minutes until vegetables are tender
~ serve hot

Blackcurrants

Blackcurrant juice is probably one of the healthiest drinks you can produce from your garden, especially for the children. There are other great things you can do with blackcurrants, too.

BLACKCURRANT JAM

ingredients
4 lbs., 1.8 kg. or 16 cups blackcurrants
3 pt., 1.7 litres or 7-1/2 cups water
6 lb., 2.7 kg. or 12 cups sugar
This quantity makes about 10 lbs. of jam (4.5 kg.). Prepare jars in advance.

method
~ prepare fruit: remove any leaves, stalks and damaged fruit
~ wash under running water and drain
~ place fruit in a large, heavy-based or preserving pan, with the water
~ bring to the boil then lower the heat and simmer for about 40–50 minutes
~ stir from time to time to prevent sticking
~ make sure the fruit is very tender and the contents have been reduced

~ remove from heat and stir in the sugar
~ keep stirring until sugar is dissolved
~ return to heat and boil rapidly for about ten minutes

Test for a set: insert a sugar thermometer into jam. When the temperature is 221F or 105C the jam is ready. Remove any scum from the surface, leave to stand for 15 minutes, then spoon the jam into prepared jars. Make sure the jars are warm before putting hot jam into them or the glass may crack.

BLACKCURRANT TART

ingredients

1 lb., 450 g. or 4 cups blackcurrants
3 oz., 75 g. or 1/3 cup sugar
4 oz. or 100 g. pastry crust
a little milk or beaten egg to glaze

method

~ preheat oven to 400F, 200C or gas mark 6
~ wash and prepare fruit
~ put a little water in a baking dish to just cover the base to prevent the fruit from sticking
~ put in half the fruit, sprinkle sugar over the top and then add the remaining fruit
~ cover with pastry crust and brush with milk or beaten egg to glaze
~ bake for about 45–50 minutes
~ cover loosely with silver (aluminium) foil to prevent over-browning

Pastry crust:

ingredients

4 oz., 100 g. or 1 cup flour
2 oz., 50 g. or 1/4 cup chilled butter
cold water

method

~ cut butter into small cubes and rub with fingertips into the flour until it resembles breadcrumbs
~ add a little cold water at a time and press dough together until it forms a smooth ball
~ knead and roll out to required size

BLACKCURRANT CREAM DESSERT

ingredients

10 oz., 250 g. or 2-1/2 cups blackcurrants
juice of half an orange
3 oz., 75 g. or 1/2 cup icing sugar
1/2 pt., 300 ml. or 1 cup whipping cream

method

~ cook fruit and orange juice until tender
~ puree in a blender or push through a sieve
~ stir in the icing sugar
~ whip the cream and fold into the puree
~ put the mixture into a freezer container
~ cover with cling film and freeze until firm

BLACKCURRANT SYRUP

ingredients

4 lbs., 1.8 kg. or 16 cups blackcurrants
grated rind and juice of 2 oranges
2 pt., 1 litre or 5 cups water
approx. 1-1/2 lbs., 675 g. or 3 cups sugar

method

~ put blackcurrants in a pan with water, orange rind and juice
~ bring to the boil, stirring constantly and boil for 2 minutes
~ remove from heat and crush blackcurrants with a wooden spoon or potato masher
~ strain through a jelly bag or a piece of muslin in a colander, into a bowl
~ pour into a measuring jug
~ weigh or measure 12 oz., 350 g. or 1-1/2 cups of sugar per pint of juice
~ put juice and sugar back in the pan and reheat, stirring constantly, until the sugar dissolves
~ bottle and sterilise by heat processing, or cool and freeze in ice cube trays or freezer bags
~ use syrup to pour over desserts, or dilute and drink as a juice

Broad Beans

Broad beans are so good for you, you should eat them with everything! Steam or boil fresh beans lightly and serve hot with any meal. If you have dried beans, they should be soaked for four hours before cooking.

BROAD BEAN SALAD

ingredients

broad beans
1 finely chopped red pepper
1 finely chopped or grated onion or shallot
Dressing:
      6 tbsp. nut or olive oil
      2 tbsp. cider vinegar
      2 tbsp. chopped herbs

method

~ steam or boil broad beans until tender but not too soft
~ drain and allow to cool
~ mix with pepper and onion
~ beat all dressing ingredients together and stir into broad beans
~ A handful of cooked and cooled broad beans can be stirred into any salad bowl.

PASTA BEAN SALAD

ingredients

6 oz., 175 g. or about 2 cups pasta shells
4–6 oz., 100–175 g. or 1 cup shelled broad beans
1 bunch watercress
1 small carrot
preferred salad dressing

method
~ cook pasta until tender but not too soft
~ drain and rinse in cold water
~ drain again and leave to cool completely
~ steam or boil broad beans until tender
~ drain and allow to cool
~ chop watercress and grate carrot
~ mix all ingredients together in a large bowl or serving dish
~ add salad dressing and serve

Broad Bean Soup

ingredients
I medium sized potato
I onion
a little oil or butter
vegetable or chicken stock
broad beans
seasoning (pepper, herbs)

method
~ peel and dice potato
~ finely chop onion
~ heat oil or butter in a large, heavy-based pan and gently fry potato and onion until soft
~ keep on a low heat and stir to prevent burning
~ add stock and as many beans as the pan will hold
~ bring to the boil, then reduce heat and simmer for 20–30 minutes until beans are soft
~ season to taste, with a little black pepper or a handful of fresh chopped herbs, or both

For non-vegetarians, add a little chopped, cooked bacon in the last five minutes of cooking.

Broad Bean Pate

ingredients
2 lb., 900 g. or 5 cups broad beans, shelled
2 tsp. ground coriander (cilantro)
2 tsp. ground parsley
2 cloves garlic, crushed
about 4 tbsp. olive oil

method
~ cook beans until tender
~ drain, reserving the liquid
~ blend beans and spices in a liquidiser (blender) or food processor
~ add garlic
~ thin the mixture with a little of the liquid to make a thick puree
~ slowly stir in the oil until the required thickness of pate is reached
~ taste and stir in a little seasoning if needed
~ serve on toast or crackers

Broccoli

BROCCOLI WITH ALMONDS

ingredients

1-1/2 lbs., 700 g. or 4 cups broccoli florets
2 oz., 50 g. or 1/4 cup butter
2 oz., 50 g. or 1/4 cup flaked or slivered almonds
a little black pepper

method

~ steam broccoli until tender and drain well
~ put into a warm serving dish
~ melt butter in a pan and gently cook almonds for about 5 minutes until they are golden
~ add a little black pepper and spoon over the broccoli

BROCCOLI IN CHEESE SAUCE

ingredients

broccoli florets
cheese sauce:
    1 oz., 25 g. or 1/4 cup flour
    1 oz., 25 g. or 2 tbsp. butter
    1/2 pt., 300 ml. or 1-1/4 cups milk
    2 oz., 50 g. or 1/2 cup finely grated hard cheese
    seasoning

method

~ steam or boil broccoli until just cooked
~ drain and place in an ovenproof serving dish
~ melt butter in a pan and stir in the flour
~ stir over a low heat for a few seconds
~ remove the pan from the heat and very slowly stir in the milk
~ return to the heat and bring to the boil
~ reduce heat and simmer for 2 or 3 minutes until sauce thickens
~ stir continuously to prevent lumps forming
~ remove from heat, season and quickly stir in grated cheese
~ stir until cheese is melted
~ pour over broccoli and grill under a moderate heat for a few minutes to brown
~ dish can also be placed in a warm oven for 10 minutes

BROCCOLI SOUP

ingredients

3 broccoli heads
1 fennel bulb
2–3 tbsp. chopped sage
vegetable or chicken stock

method

~ cut fennel into small pieces
~ bring stock to the boil in a fairly large pan and add fennel
~ reduce heat and simmer for about 10 minutes
~ separate broccoli florets and cut stems into thin slices
~ add all the broccoli to the pan with the sage and simmer for a further 10–15 minutes until all vegetables are tender

~ blend in a liquidiser (blender) or food processor and serve in warm bowls with croutons or crusty bread

BROCCOLI QUICHE

ingredients

handful of broccoli florets
2 beaten eggs
5 fl. oz., 150 ml. or 1/2 cup milk or single cream
4 oz., 100 g. or 1 cup hard cheese, grated
seasoning
pastry crust, bought or made with:
      6 oz., 150 g. or 1-1/2 cups flour
      3 oz., 75 g. or 6 tbsp. butter
      cold water

method

To make your own pastry crust:
~ cut butter into small cubes and rub with fingertips into the flour until it resembles breadcrumbs
~ add a little cold water at a time and press dough together until it forms a smooth ball
~ knead for a few minutes
~ roll out pastry and line a lightly greased, deep ovenproof dish
~ cover pastry base with a circle of greaseproof (wax) paper and scatter a handful of dried beans on top
~ bake in a preheated oven, 400F, 200C or gas mark 6 for 10–15 minutes, until pastry is set
~ remove from oven and leave to cool slightly but keep the oven on
~ steam or boil broccoli and drain well
~ remove the beans and greaseproof paper and cover the pastry base with broccoli
~ sprinkle grated cheese over the broccoli
~ beat the eggs together with the milk or cream and season
~ pour over the broccoli and cheese and bake in the oven for about 30 minutes until golden brown in colour

Cabbage

There are many recipes for cabbage, from cold, summer dishes to warm and welcoming winter soups and stews.

CABBAGE SOUP

ingredients

1 white cabbage
2 stalks celery
1 onion
2 carrots
vegetable or chicken stock
2 or 3 bay leaves
handful of chopped parsley

method

seasoning
cooking oil or butter
~ finely slice the celery, onion and carrots
~ heat the oil or melt the butter in a large pan and gently cook the celery, onion and carrots for about 5 minutes
~ add the stock, bay leaves and parsley to the pan and bring to the boil
~ shred the cabbage finely and add to the pan
~ cover and simmer for about 40–50 minutes until all vegetables are tender
~ remove the bay leaves and add seasoning to taste

COLE SLAW

ingredients

1 white cabbage finely shredded OR
1 green cabbage, shredded, steamed, drained and left to cool
1 grated onion
handful of chopped walnuts or pecan nuts
1 apple, peeled, cored and grated
4 level tbsp. mayonnaise
4 level tbsp. natural yoghurt

method

~ mix cabbage, onion, apple and nuts in a bowl or serving dish
~ stir mayonnaise and natural yoghurt together and mix into the vegetables
~ chill before serving

NUTTY CABBAGE

ingredients

finely sliced cabbage
a little butter
a handful of chopped mixed nuts

method

~ steam or boil cabbage until tender
~ drain well
~ melt a little butter and mix into the cabbage with nuts
~ serve hot as a side vegetable

BAKED CABBAGE

ingredients

1 green or white cabbage
4 ripe chopped tomatoes, or 1 can chopped tomatoes
4–5 tbsp. of chicken or vegetable stock
1 tsp. paprika or preferred spice
a little olive oil
3 firm tomatoes for topping
black pepper

method

~ preheat oven to 350F, 180C or gas mark 4
~ shred the whole cabbage
~ heat a little olive oil and water in a large frying pan and gently cook the cabbage for about 10 minutes, stirring occasionally
~ add stock, chopped tomatoes and paprika and cook for another 10 minutes
~ spread the mixture into an ovenproof dish

~ slice the firm tomatoes and arrange over the top of the cabbage
~ add black pepper and brush the whole surface with a little olive oil
~ cook for 30–40 minutes in preheated oven until tomatoes are just starting to brown
~ serve hot, garnished with a little parsley or basil

Carrots

Carrots can be eaten in so many different ways, there is bound to be some tasty way you can incorporate them into your healthy diet.

GARLIC CARROTS

ingredients

carrots
1–2 cloves garlic, crushed or finely chopped
a little butter
1 tbsp. chopped, fresh parsley

method

~ scrub carrots and slice into circles or fine sticks
~ steam until just cooked
~ drain and toss in butter, garlic, and parsley
~ stir gently and serve immediately

CARROT, ORANGE AND ALMOND SOUP

ingredients

6 carrots sliced
2 onions chopped
2 pts., 1 litre or 5 cups vegetable or chicken stock
4 oz., 100 g. or 2/3 cup ground almonds
1 orange
a little butter
seasoning

method

~ melt the butter in a large pan and add the prepared carrots and onions
~ cook gently for a few minutes until vegetables begin to soften, don't let it burn
~ add the stock and seasoning to taste and bring to the boil
~ reduce heat and simmer for about 40 minutes until vegetables are tender
~ allow the soup to cool slightly, then blend in a liquidiser (blender) or food processor
~ return to the pan
~ finely grate half the peel from the orange and add to the soup with the ground almonds
~ squeeze the juice from the orange and add to the pan
~ reheat gently for a few minutes and serve hot

CARROT CAKE

ingredients

8 oz., 200 g. or 2 cups flour
2 tsp. baking powder
5 oz., 125 g. or 3/4 cup sugar
2 oz., 50 g. or 1/2 cup chopped walnuts
4 carrots, grated

2 bananas, mashed
2 eggs, beaten
5 fl. oz., 150 ml. or 1/2 cup sunflower oil
1–2 tsp. mixed spice (cinnamon, nutmeg, allspice)
handful of raisins
For topping
    cream cheese
    icing sugar (powdered sugar)

method

~ preheat oven to 350F, 180C or gas mark 4
~ beat all ingredients together well and pour into a lightly greased cake pan
~ bake for about 1 hour on the centre rack of the oven
~ remove and cool thoroughly on a wire rack
~ blend cream cheese and icing sugar to make a topping and spread over cooled cake

CARROT STICKS

Carrots cut into thin sticks are popular and healthy snacks. Very young children shouldn't be left alone with raw carrots as they can easily choke on them. It's always good to encourage children to eat healthy snacks and carrots are a tasty alternative to processed snack foods.

CARROTS FOR BULK

Scrub (or peel if non-organic) your carrots and chop into small pieces. Use to add bulk to bolognaise, shepherd's pie, lasagna and other one-pot dishes. Chopped carrots can also be added to beef or chicken stews and soups.

JUST-COOKED CARROTS

Thin carrot sticks can be stir-fried along with bean shoots (sprouts), peppers, mushrooms and any other fresh vegetables you have available. They will stay crisp and add a crunch to your stir-fry that is very appealing and colourful.

Cauliflower

Raw cauliflower florets make great, crunchy, healthy snacks. A medium sized cauliflower with a cheese sauce is enough to make a main meal for a family of four.

CRISPY CAULIFLOWER SALAD

ingredients

1 medium cauliflower
1 apple, cored and diced
a handful of chopped walnuts or pecans
1 tbsp. lemon juice
2 hardboiled eggs, shelled and chopped

method

~ break cauliflower into small florets
~ toss apple pieces in lemon juice
~ mix cauliflower and apple together in a bowl or serving dish
~ add walnuts and egg and stir gently together
~ season and serve with preferred salad dressing, mayonnaise or natural yoghurt

CURRIED CAULIFLOWER

ingredients

I medium cauliflower, broken into florets
I onion, peeled and chopped
curry sauce
a little cooking oil

method

~ preheat oven to 350F, 180C or gas mark 4
~ heat the cooking oil in a wok or large frying pan and gently cook cauliflower
  and onion for a few minutes, stirring to prevent burning
~ put vegetables into an ovenproof dish and cover with curry sauce
~ cook in oven for 30–40 minutes until cauliflower is tender
~ serve hot on a bed of rice or with jacket potatoes (baked potatoes)

CAULIFLOWER AND LEEK SOUP

ingredients

I cauliflower broken into florets
2 onions, peeled and chopped
2–3 celery stalks, finely sliced
3 leeks, trimmed and thinly sliced
a little olive oil
vegetable or chicken stock

method

~ heat oil in a large pan and cook all vegetables for a few minutes
~ add stock and bring to the boil
~ reduce heat and simmer for 20–30 minutes or until the vegetables are tender
~ cool for 5 minutes then blend in a liquidiser (blender) or food processor
~ heat gently for a few minutes, adding a little water if needed
~ serve hot

STIR FRIED CAULIFLOWER AND CARROTS

ingredients

I cauliflower, broken into florets
6 carrots, sliced into rings or short sticks
I–2 cloves garlic, crushed
3 or 4 spring onions, or 2 small shallots, chopped
olive oil
I–2 tbsp. soy sauce (tamari)

method

~ put cauliflower and carrots into a pan and cover with water
~ bring to the boil and simmer for 3 minutes
~ drain well
~ heat oil in a wok or large frying pan
~ add garlic, onions and soy sauce and cook for I minute, stirring to prevent
  burning
~ add carrots and cauliflower and stir fry for about 2 or 3 minutes
~ serve hot.

Celeriac

Celeriac is a wholesome root vegetable with a strong, celery flavour and can be eaten raw or cooked.

CELERIAC AND ONION BAKE

ingredients

1 celeriac root
1 large onion
2 oz., 50 g. or 2 tbsp. butter
1/4 pt., 150 ml. or 1/2 cup milk
seasoning / mixed herbs

method

~ preheat oven to 375F, 190C or gas mark 5
~ peel and thinly slice celeriac and onion and layer in an ovenproof dish
~ dot a little butter onto each layer
~ pour milk over the top and bake in a preheated oven for 1 to 1-1/2 hours, or until tender and golden brown
~ serve hot

CELERIAC SALAD

ingredients

1 celeriac root
1 tbsp. wine or cider vinegar
a little salt
3 tbsp. mayonnaise
3 tbsp. natural yoghurt
1 tbsp. French (Dijon) mustard

method

~ peel celeriac
~ cut into very fine strips or grate
~ put into a bowl and cover with water
~ add vinegar and a little salt and leave to soak for 15–20 minutes
~ drain and blanch celeriac in boiling water for about 15 seconds
~ drain, rinse under cold water, drain again and cool
~ mix together mayonnaise, yoghurt and mustard and stir into the celeriac
~ chill before serving

STUFFED CELERIAC

ingredients

4 small celeriac roots
juice of 2 lemons
1/4 pt., 150 ml. or 1/2 cup olive oil
6 cloves of garlic, finely chopped
1–2 tsp freshly ground black pepper
5–6 tbsp. chopped parsley

method

~ peel celeriac and immerse in a bowl of water
~ add lemon juice
~ lift out the celeriac one by one and carefully scoop out the flesh leaving a shell about 1/2 to 1 inch thick
~ put all celeriac flesh in a large bowl and mix with garlic, parsley and pepper

~ spoon the stuffing back into the celeriac shells and place them in a large pan, making sure they won't fall over during cooking

~ pour in the olive oil and some of the lemon water to about halfway up the celeriac

~ cover, bring to the boil then reduce heat and simmer very gently for about 30 minutes

~ when the celeriac is tender and nearly all liquid has been absorbed, carefully remove from pan and serve hot or cold

Duchesse Potatoes with Celeriac

ingredients

1 lb., 450 g. or about 2-1/2 cups potatoes, peeled and cut into cubes
8 oz., 225 g. or about 1-1/2 cups celeriac, peeled and cut into cubes
1 oz., 25 g. or 2 tbsp. butter
squeeze of lemon juice
1 egg, beaten
seasoning

method

~ preheat oven to 400F, 200C or gas mark 6

~ boil potatoes and celeriac together with the lemon juice until soft but not mushy

~ drain well, then add butter and seasoning and mash until smooth

~ cool slightly then add beaten egg and mix well

~ place in spoonfuls on a greased baking tray and bake for about 20 minutes until golden

~ serve hot

Chicory

Chicory root has been roasted, ground and used as a healthy substitute for coffee for many generations. The rest of the plant is just as useful.

Baked Chicory in Parsley Sauce

ingredients

4 chicory heads
1 oz., 25 g. or 2 tbsp. butter
juice of half a lemon
1/4 pt., 150 ml., or 1/2 cup chicken or vegetable stock
Parsley sauce
    1 oz., 25 g. or 1/4 cup flour
    1 oz., 25 g. or 2 tbsp butter
    1/2 pt., 300 ml. or 1 cup milk
    handful of fresh parsley, chopped
    seasoning

method

~ preheat oven to 325F, 170C or gas mark 3

~ trim and wash chicory

~ blanch in boiling water for a minute or two

~ drain, rinse in cold water and drain again

~ place in an ovenproof dish and dot with butter

~ mix lemon juice with stock and pour over chicory

~ cover and cook in preheated oven for about 1-1/2 hours until chicory is tender

~ drain the juice

To make the sauce:

~ melt butter in a pan and stir in the flour

~ stir over a low heat for a few seconds

~ remove the pan from the heat and very slowly stir in the milk

~ return to the heat and bring to the boil

~ reduce heat and simmer for 2 or 3 minutes until sauce thickens

~ stir continuously to prevent lumps forming

~ remove from heat, season and stir in parsley

~ arrange chicory on a serving dish and pour the parsley sauce over it

~ serve immediately

FRUITY CHICORY SALAD

ingredients

2 chicory heads, trimmed and sliced

1 small grapefruit

2 oranges

3 or 4 tomatoes, peeled and chopped

Dressing

    3 tbsp. nut oil

    1 tbsp. lemon juice

    2–4 tsp. brown sugar

    handful of chopped fresh herbs

method

~ peel and remove pith and seeds from grapefruit and oranges

~ cut into segments and place in salad bowl

~ add sliced chicory and peeled, chopped tomatoes and gently stir all ingredients together

~ whisk dressing ingredients together and pour over salad

CHICORY AND FRESH TOMATO SAUCE

ingredients

4 chicory heads

1 onion, peeled and chopped

1 garlic clove, finely chopped

6 ripe tomatoes, skinned and chopped

1 bay leaf

1 sprig of thyme

a handful of fresh basil, chopped

dash of white wine

1 oz., 25 g. or about 1/4 cup fresh parmesan, grated

1 tbsp. olive oil

method

~ heat oil in a pan, and gently cook onions and garlic for 5 minutes

~ add tomatoes, bay leaf and thyme

~ stir and simmer for 15 minutes, stirring occasionally to prevent sticking

~ remove bay leaf and thyme

~ add wine and chopped basil and simmer for a further 5 minutes

~ cook chicory in boiling water until tender, adding a little salt to the water if desired

~ drain well and place chicory in a ovenproof dish

~ cover with the tomato sauce

~ sprinkle on the grated cheese and grill for a few minutes until sauce starts to bubble

~ serve immediately

CHICORY TART

ingredients

6 oz. readymade pastry crust (or make your own, see below)

8 oz., 200 g. or 1 cup soft cream cheese

1/4 pint, 150 ml. or 1/2 cup single cream

3 heads chicory

2 large eggs, beaten

a little grated nutmeg

seasoning

method

~ preheat oven to 400F, 200C or gas mark 6

~ boil chicory until tender

~ drain well, cool then chop

~ line an ovenproof dish with pastry

~ mix cheese in a bowl until smooth

~ add eggs and beat well

~ mix in chicory, cream, nutmeg and seasoning

~ pour into pastry and bake for about 35 minutes until set and lightly browned

ingredients

To make your own pastry crust you will need:

  6 oz., 150 g. or 1-1/2 cups flour

  3 oz., 50 g. or just under 1/2 cup chilled butter

  cold water

method

~ cut butter into small cubes and rub with fingertips into the flour until it resembles breadcrumbs

~ add a little cold water at a time and press dough together until it forms a smooth ball

~ knead for a few minutes and roll out to required size

Cos Lettuce

Cos or romaine lettuce is a versatile salad vegetable with large leaves and lots of them!

EVERYDAY SALAD

ingredients

1 cos lettuce
3 or 4 spring onions or 1 small onion
1 green pepper
handful of walnuts or pecans
1 tomato if desired
Vinaigrette Dressing
> olive oil
> wine or cider vinegar
> mustard
> seasoning

method

~ finely slice all vegetables and mix together in a large bowl or serving dish
~ stir in the nuts and chill for a few minutes before serving
~ whisk all dressing ingredients together
~ add a little more oil if too acidic and adjust seasoning to taste
~ toss salad in vinaigrette dressing and serve immediately

LETTUCE SOUP

ingredients

12 oz., 350 g. or 4 cups cos lettuce leaves, chopped
1 pt., 500–600 ml. or 2-1/2 cups vegetable or chicken stock
1 level tbsp. flour
2 oz., 50 g. or 1/4 cup butter
4 oz., 125 g. or 1 cup spring onions, or shallots, sliced
1/4 pt., 150 ml. or 1/2 cup milk
seasoning

method

~ melt butter in a large pan
~ add lettuce and onions and cook gently until soft, stirring to prevent burning
~ stir in the flour and add stock
~ bring to the boil, reduce heat and simmer for about 20 minutes
~ cool for 5–10 minutes, then blend in a liquidiser (blender) or food processor until smooth
~ return to the pan, add milk and seasoning and reheat gently
~ serve hot with crusty bread or croutons

BOILED EGG AND LETTUCE SALAD

ingredients

1 cos lettuce
2–3 hardboiled eggs
3 tbsp. mayonnaise
3 tbsp. natural yoghurt
handful of chopped chives or finely chopped spring onion

method

~ prepare the lettuce and arrange on a serving dish
~ peel and chop hardboiled eggs in a bowl and stir in chives or onions
~ spoon egg mixture onto lettuce leaves
~ mix together the mayonnaise and yoghurt and spoon over the egg mixture
~ serve chilled

Sandwiches and Salads

Lettuce can be added to practically any sandwich and forms the base for many different salads. Shred finely and add to chicken sandwiches or make a Caesar Salad by adding hot sliced chicken to a bed of torn lettuce leaves. Toss in a garlic and olive oil dressing. Add lettuce to bacon and tomato and serve with whole grain bread as an open sandwich. Slice lettuce finely and lay slices of boiled egg in a wholemeal bread sandwich.

Courgettes

When the courgettes get going in the garden you won't be able to eat them fast enough. Serve them in as many different ways as possible.

Courgettes with Herbs

ingredients

1-1/2 lbs., 750 g. or 3 cups courgettes, cut into fairly thin slices
1 oz., 25 g. or 2 tbsp. butter
handful of fresh chopped herbs
seasoning

method

~ put the courgette slices into a large pan and cover with water
~ bring to the boil, reduce heat and simmer for about five minutes, until tender
~ drain well and return to the pan
~ add butter, herbs and a little seasoning and stir well
~ serve hot

Courgette Pasta Salad

ingredients

4 courgettes, cut into thin slices
2 tomatoes, chopped
3–4 spring onions, or 2 shallots
1 tbsp. chopped parsley
1–2 cloves garlic, finely chopped or crushed
6 oz., 175 g. or about 2 cups pasta shells
seasoning
preferred salad dressing

method

~ put the courgette slices into a large pan and cover with water
~ bring to the boil, reduce heat and simmer for about five minutes, until tender
~ cool
~ cook the pasta shells in boiling water and drain well
~ mix a little salad dressing into the pasta and leave to cool
~ chop tomatoes and onions
~ when pasta and courgettes are cool mix all ingredients together
~ chill for 10 minutes or more before serving

Stuffed Courgettes

ingredients

8 large courgettes
1 large onion, finely chopped
1 ripe tomato, finely chopped
2–4 oz., 50–100 g. or 1/2 to 1 cup grated hard cheese

4 oz ., 100 g. or 1 cup sliced mushrooms
handful of sweet corn kernels
1 egg, beaten
seasoning

method

~ heat oven to 350F, 180C or gas mark 4
~ blanch the courgettes in boiling water for about 3 minutes
~ drain and allow to cool a little
~ cut in half lengthwise and scoop out the seeds leaving a hollow in each courgette
~ mix the rest of the ingredients together and pile into the courgette hollows
~ place the courgettes, stuffing side up, into a shallow, greased, ovenproof dish
~ bake for 30–40 minutes until tender
~ serve hot

CREAMY COURGETTES

ingredients

about 1 lb., 450 g. or 3 cups courgettes, cut into thick slices
a little olive oil or other cooking oil
2–4 oz., 50–100 g. or 1/2 to 1 cup peeled almonds (soak overnight in water to peel easily)
seasoning
3 tbsp. flour
5 fl. oz., 150 ml. or 1/2 cup crème fraiche or sour cream

method

~ mix seasoning into flour
~ toss the courgette slices in the flour
~ warm a serving dish
~ heat oil in a pan and gently fry the courgette slices until golden brown
~ cook a few at a time, drain and put into warm serving dish
~ when courgettes are cooked, toss the almonds into the oil for a minute or two
~ add the crème fraiche or sour cream and stir
~ reduce heat and cook gently for a minute or two, stirring constantly
~ pour the cream and almonds over the courgettes and serve immediately

Dandelion Greens

Dandelion greens can be bitter so choose young leaves if possible or change the water during cooking. Boil for a few minutes, drain, rinse and cook in fresh water for the remainder of the cooking time. Use dandelion greens in place of spinach or any recipe needing greens.

All parts of the dandelion plant are useful and nutritious. Just be sure the area hasn't been previously treated with a herbicide that may still be in the plant.

Leaves   Use the young leaves in salads and as part of a stir fry. Serve separately with a rice dish or pasta. Dandelion greens are a useful green, leafy vegetable and can be cooked and eaten as any other greens. And if you are ever out in the wilderness without any food, dandelions may come to your rescue!

Stems The milky sap from the stem is very effective in treating warts and verrucas. Dab the sap onto the affected area a few times every day and the wart will gradually fade away. I've had great success with this natural remedy on children's verrucas.

Roots The roots can be roasted, ground and used as a coffee substitute – wonderful for getting off caffeine. The powdered root can be made into a medicine for treating premenstrual syndrome and high blood pressure. Over the centuries poultices and potions have been made from dandelions to treat many conditions, including colds, ulcers, and obesity. The dandelion is said to be helpful in dissolving gallstones and even alleviating pain due to heart conditions. Ayurvedic physicians commonly use dandelion in their preparations.

Always check with a doctor or recognised herbalist before taking any new treatments. Pregnant women shouldn't take dandelion preparations because of their diuretic properties.

Flowers Dandelion flowers can be made into a delicious jam. I used an old, traditional French recipe and tested it on the family. The 3 jars lasted 3 days. The recipe states you must make the jam in batches of 365 flowers, and yes, I did count them all! If you double the recipe it doesn't work. Simmer the flowers and make the jam as if the dandelion flowers were your fruit ingredient. Add preserving sugar, a lemon and an orange or two and simmer until at setting point. Pour into sterilised jars and label.

Fennel

The strong aniseed taste of the fennel bulb makes it a tasty addition to any salad or served as a side dish.

BRAISED FENNEL

ingredients

4 small fennel bulbs
2 carrots, sliced
2–3 stalks celery, sliced
1 onion, chopped
1 green or red pepper, sliced into rings or chopped finely
a little butter or cooking oil
about 1 pt., 500 ml. or 2-1/2 cups vegetable or chicken stock
a handful of mixed, chopped herbs

method

~ preheat oven to 350F, 180C or gas mark 4
~ heat butter or oil in a pan and gently cook carrots, onion, pepper and celery for a few minutes, stirring to prevent burning
~ put all vegetables in an ovenproof dish
~ add the herbs
~ cut the fennel bulbs in half and place, cut side down, on top of the mixed vegetables
~ pour the stock over and add a little seasoning if desired

~ bake for about an hour until fennel is tender

~ serve as it is, or remove the fennel, blend the rest of the vegetables and liquid and use as a sauce to pour over the fennel

FENNEL AND TOMATO

ingredients

1–2 fennel bulbs
2–3 ripe tomatoes
5 fl. oz., 150 ml. or 1/2 cup vegetable oil (or half olive and half walnut oil)
juice of half a lemon
black pepper

method

~ whisk oils, lemon juice and pepper together and chill slightly
~ trim and slice fennel bulbs and blanch in boiling water for 2–3 minutes
~ place on a serving dish and pour the dressing over the fennel while it is still warm
~ cool completely and add thinly sliced tomatoes to the dish just before serving

FENNEL AND ORANGE

ingredients

1 fennel bulb
2 oranges
lettuce leaves
3 tbsp. olive oil
1–2 tbsp. lemon juice
1 clove of garlic, crushed
black pepper
1 tbsp. fresh parsley, chopped

method

~ remove all peel and pith from the oranges
~ slice in rounds and remove any pips (seeds)
~ slice the fennel
~ arrange oranges, fennel and lettuce leaves in a serving dish
~ whisk together the oil, lemon juice, garlic, pepper and parsley and pour over the salad
~ chill slightly before serving
~ to decorate the salad, cut very fine strips of orange peel, removing any white pith, and toss them into the salad

FENNEL SOUP

ingredients

3 fennel bulbs
2 celery stalks
1 small onion
a handful of chopped fresh herbs
a little cooking oil
2 pints, 1 litre or 5 cups vegetable or chicken stock
a little single cream (optional)

method

~ finely slice fennel, celery and onion
~ heat the oil in a large pan and cook the vegetables for a few minutes
~ add herbs and pour in the stock

~ bring to the boil, reduce heat and simmer for about 20 minutes until tender
~ serve as a clear soup or cool slightly and blend in a liquidiser (blender) or food processor until smooth
~ reheat gently for a few minutes
~ pour into warm serving bowls and swirl a little single cream into each bowl if desired

Garlic

Garlic is a powerful cleanser and can be safely added, in moderation, to the daily diet. To avoid 'garlic breath', chew on a few parsley leaves after your meal.

GARLIC CARROTS

ingredients

carrots
1–2 cloves garlic
a little butter

method

~ peel and slice carrots into rings or thin sticks
~ steam for about 10 minutes until just cooked
~ drain well and return to the pan
~ crush or finely chop garlic and sprinkle over the carrots
~ add a little butter and stir gently until melted
~ serve hot

GARLIC BREAD

ingredients

1 large French loaf
6 oz., 175 g. or 3/4 cup butter
3–4 cloves garlic, crushed
1 tbsp. fresh parsley, chopped

method

~ preheat oven to 350F, 180C or gas mark 4
~ slice loaf into 1 inch (2.5 cm.) thick slices
~ soften the butter and beat with the garlic and parsley
~ spread on every cut surface of the bread and place slices together to re-form the loaf
~ wrap loosely in foil and bake in the oven for about 15–20 minutes
~ serve hot

GARLIC MASH

ingredients

mashed potato
cooked bacon, cut into small pieces
3 cloves garlic, crushed
1 tbsp. fresh parsley, chopped
a little butter

method

~ preheat oven to 350F, 180C or gas mark 4
~ mix mashed potato in a bowl with the cooked bacon pieces, garlic and parsley
~ lightly grease an ovenproof dish with butter and spread the potato mix into it

~ bake in the oven until thoroughly hot (around 20–30 minutes)

~ sprinkle a little grated cheese on top and place under a grill (broiler) for 1–2 minutes if desired

ROAST GARLIC SALAD

ingredients

6–8 cloves garlic, left in their skin
a little cooking oil
young spinach or lettuce leaves
1 firm tomato, chopped
1/4 cucumber, chopped
Dressing
     3 tbsp. olive or nut oil
     1 tbsp. lemon juice
     1 tbsp. fresh, finely chopped herbs
     black pepper

method

~ preheat oven to 375F, 190C or gas mark 5

~ put all garlic cloves in a roasting pan and pour a little cooking oil over them

~ bake for about 15 minutes until the cloves look a little brown round the edge

~ while they are still warm, put them into a salad bowl and add the remaining ingredients whisk together the dressing ingredients, pour over the salad and toss well

~ squeeze the garlic out of their skins to eat

Green Beans

Green beans will produce more beans than you can possibly use when they get going. Make the most of them and freeze a few for the winter months.

GREEN BEANS WITH GARLIC AND BASIL

ingredients

1 lb., 450 g. or about 2-1/2 cups green beans
2 garlic cloves, chopped
1 tbsp. basil, chopped
2 tbsp. olive oil
black pepper

method

~ cook beans in boiling water until just tender

~ drain well

~ heat the oil in a large frying pan or wok

~ cook garlic for a minute then add beans, basil and black pepper

~ stir and heat thoroughly

~ serve immediately

GREEN BEAN SALAD

ingredients

1 lb., 450 g. or about 2-1/2 cups young green beans
4 oz., 100 g. or 1 cup feta cheese, cut or crumbled into small pieces
1 tbsp. pitted, black olives
1 small lettuce

1 handful of watercress
1 tbsp. chopped chives
1 handful of young spinach leaves
vinaigrette dressing or dressing of choice

method

~ cook beans until just tender, drain well and cool completely
~ arrange leaves in a serving dish
~ place beans, feta cheese and olives on top
~ sprinkle on chives and pour over vinaigrette dressing just before serving

Green Beans with Sour Cream and Almonds

ingredients

1 lb., 450 g. or about 2-1/2 cups green beans
3 oz., 75 g. or 1 cup flaked or sliced almonds (or mushrooms)
1 oz., 25 g. or 2 tbsp. butter
2–3 fl. oz., 75 ml. or 1/4 cup sour cream
1 tsp. oregano chopped

method

~ steam beans until tender
~ drain well
~ heat butter in a large frying pan or wok and gently brown the almonds
~ add beans and oregano and heat thoroughly
~ stir in sour cream and serve immediately

Green Beans and Thyme

ingredients

1-1/2 lbs., 700 g. or 4 cups green beans, trimmed and prepared
1 onion, peeled and sliced finely
1 oz., 25 g. or 2 tbsp. butter
1 tsp. fresh thyme, chopped
6 tbsp. or 90 ml. vegetable or ham stock
seasoning

method

~ melt butter in a large saucepan and cook onion until it starts to change colour
~ add beans, thyme, seasoning and stock
~ bring to the boil, lower heat, cover and simmer for about 10 minutes until
   beans are cooked but still a little crisp
~ serve immediately

Hazelnuts

If you don't have a nut allergy, nuts are a great source of protein and make a good alternative to eating meat or fish – perfect for vegetarians.

Straight from the shell

Most nuts are harvested in the late summer or autumn and store well during the winter months. A bowl of mixed nuts is part of the décor in many homes throughout the Thanksgiving and Christmas periods. Enjoy the taste and eat a few different varieties of nuts every day. Never eat too many as your digestive system will be put under a lot of stress in dealing with them.

ROASTED

Shell and lightly roast hazelnuts.

SALADS

Throw a handful of any shelled nuts into the salad bowl.

BLANCHED

Remove hard shells and blanch by plunging into boiling water. Remove inner skin so you are left with the clean, white nut. Blend in a food blender and use in any number of delicious recipes.

DECORATION

Blanched, halved almonds, walnuts, pecans and hazelnuts are all used to decorate speciality cakes and gateaux. A few whole nuts decorating the simplest of dishes can turn them into cordon bleu creations.

HAZELNUT COOKIES

ingredients

6 oz., 150 g. or 1-1/2 cups ground toasted hazelnuts
6 oz., 150 g. or 1 cup firm raw brown sugar
1 egg, beaten
a little cooking oil

method

~ preheat oven to 350F, 180C or gas mark 4
~ mix the nuts, sugar and egg together
~ oil a surface and a rolling pin and roll out the dough to a thin layer
~ cut into rounds and place on greaseproof (wax) paper on a baking sheet
~ cook in the oven for about 10 minutes or until golden in colour
~ cool on a wire rack

HAZELNUT CAKES

Use any favourite sponge cake recipe and replace 1 or 2 oz., 25–50 g. or 1/4 to 1/2 cup flour with ground hazelnuts. Add some ground hazelnuts to the filling and decorate with a few whole nuts to finish.

Kale

Kale is a wonderful stand by green vegetable throughout the winter months, however, it can be a little bitter. To get around the bitter taste cook it for a few minutes then change the water and finish cooking in fresh water.

KALE SOUP

ingredients

8 oz., 200 g. or 2 cups kale, chopped
1 onion, chopped
1–2 cloves of garlic, crushed
2 turnips or carrots, peeled and chopped
1-1/2 pints, 750 ml. or 3-3/4 cups vegetable or chicken stock
handful of fresh, chopped herbs
seasoning

method

a little cooking oil

~ heat oil in a large pan and gently cook the onion, garlic and turnips/carrots for a few minutes

~ add the stock and bring to the boil

~ reduce heat and simmer for about 15 minutes

~ add the chopped kale and herbs and cook for a further 10–15 minutes until all vegetables are tender

~ add seasoning

~ allow to cool and blend in a liquidiser (blender) or food processor until smooth

~ return to pan and reheat gently for a few minutes

~ serve hot

KALE AND POTATO CAKES

ingredients

8 oz., 225 g. or 2 cups kale

1 lb., 450 g. or 2 cups mashed potato

2 eggs, beaten

2 oz., 50 g. or 1 cup breadcrumbs

2 oz., 50 g., or 1/4 cup butter (or 2 tbsp. sunflower oil)

1 onion, chopped

seasoning

method

~ cut out coarse ribs from middle of kale leaves, shred and put into a pan of boiling water for 2 minutes

~ drain thoroughly and allow to cool

~ saute chopped onion until golden brown

~ put kale, potato, eggs, breadcrumbs, seasoning and onion into a bowl and mix together

~ form into small cakes and chill in the fridge for about 30 minutes

~ cook in butter or oil for 7 or 8 minutes, turning occasionally, until crispy

BEAN AND KALE SOUP

ingredients

2 pints, 1 litre or 5 cups chicken or vegetable stock

8 oz., 225 g. or just over 1 cup cannelloni beans

2 onions, chopped

1 carrot, chopped

2 sticks celery, chopped

1 lb., 450 g. or 2-1/4 cups ripe tomatoes, skinned and chopped or 1 tin plum tomatoes

8 oz., 225 g. or 2 cups kale, shredded

3 cloves garlic, chopped

2 oz., 50 g. or 1/4 cup smoked bacon (optional)

1 tbsp. olive oil

handful of fresh chopped herbs

1–2 tbsp. grated parmesan

1 large sprig of thyme, 1 sprig of rosemary and 1 bay leaf tied together in a bunch

method

~ soak cannelloni beans overnight, rinse, put in a large pan and cover with water
~ bring to the boil, skim off any scum and then boil rapidly for 10 minutes
~ lower the heat and simmer until almost cooked
~ drain and rinse
~ heat oil in a large pan and gently saute onion and garlic
~ add chopped bacon and cook for a few more minutes
~ add celery, carrot, tomatoes and the bunch of herbs
~ mix in beans and stock and bring to the boil
~ lower heat and simmer for 40 minutes
~ add kale and simmer until kale is cooked
~ remove the bunch of herbs
~ serve piping hot, sprinkled with fresh chopped herbs and parmesan

STIR-FRIED KALE

ingredients

1 lb., 450 g. or 4 cups kale
1 onion, chopped
1/2 inch or 1 to 1-1/2 cm. fresh ginger, chopped
2 cloves of garlic, chopped
2 tbsp. olive or nut oil
1 tsp. soy sauce or tamari
1 tbsp. chives, chopped
1/2 tsp. Chinese spice (if available)

method

~ cut out ribs from kale leaves, shred and cook in boiling water for 2 or 3 minutes
~ drain well
~ heat oil in a large frying pan or wok
~ gently saute onion, garlic, ginger and spice
~ add cooked kale
~ stir together and heat thoroughly
~ sprinkle with soy sauce and chives
~ serve immediately

Mushrooms

Mushrooms can be eaten in so many ways. You're only limited in recipes by your imagination.

MUSHROOM OMELETTE

To make one omelette:

ingredients

2 eggs
2 oz., 50 g. or 2/3 cup sliced mushrooms
a little cooking oil
seasoning
a little grated cheese (optional)

method

~ heat oil in a frying pan and add sliced mushrooms
~ cook gently for a few minutes
~ beat the eggs well and add to the pan
~ cook for a couple of minutes
~ turn the whole omelette over and cook for a couple of minutes on the other side
~ add seasoning and cheese just before serving
~ serve hot with a green salad

Garlic Mushrooms

ingredients

1–2 cloves garlic, crushed
1–2 oz., 25–50 g. or 2–4 tbsp. butter
small, whole mushrooms

method

~ heat butter in a pan and add garlic
~ stir and add mushrooms
~ gently stir over a low heat for a few minutes until hot

Mushroom Scramble

ingredients

To serve one:
2 eggs, lightly beaten
seasoning
a little grated hard cheese
2–3 mushrooms, finely chopped
1 tsp. mustard
a little butter

method

~ add cheese, mushrooms, mustard and seasoning to lightly beaten eggs
~ heat butter in a saucepan and pour in the egg mixture
~ with a wooden spoon, stir over a very low heat until the eggs are set
~ serve immediately on hot buttered toast

Mushroom Sauce

ingredients

1 oz., 25 g. or 1/4 cup flour
1 oz., 25 g. or 2 tbsp. butter
1/2 pt., 300 ml. or 1-1/4 cup milk
handful of finely chopped, fresh mushrooms
seasoning

method

~ melt butter in a pan and mix in the flour
~ with a wire whisk, stir over a low heat for a few seconds
~ remove the pan from the heat and very slowly stir in the milk
~ return to the heat and bring to the boil
~ reduce heat and simmer for 2 or 3 minutes until sauce thickens
~ stir or whisk continuously to prevent lumps forming
~ add mushrooms and cook for a few seconds, stirring continuously

MUSHROOM IDEAS

- Veggie alternative: use firm, white mushrooms in place of chicken in recipes that require cut chicken, such as curries and stir-frys.
- Make a creamy mushroom soup.
- Add to ratatouille or add raw, sliced mushrooms to the salad bowl.
- Stuffed mushrooms: make a sage and onion stuffing mix, remove stems from large mushrooms and place a spoonful of the stuffing on the underside the mushrooms. Sprinkle a little grated cheese on top and place stuffing side up in a lightly greased baking dish. Bake in a moderate oven for about 20 minutes.
- Dip small, firm mushrooms in a coating batter and deep fry for a minute or two – naughty but very tasty!

nions

A kitchen should never be without onions. Apart from being very good for you, they will make any meal tastier.

FRENCH ONION SOUP

ingredients

3 oz., 75 g. or 6 tbsp. butter
1-1/2 to 2 lbs., 750–900 g. or 6–8 cups onions, sliced
1 tbsp. flour
seasoning
2 pts., 1 litre or 5 cups preferred stock (vegetable, chicken or beef)

method

~ melt the butter in a large pan and add the onions
~ cook gently for a few minutes until the onions are soft and golden brown in colour
~ stir in the flour and gradually add stock, stirring continuously
~ add seasoning and bring to the boil
~ reduce heat and simmer for about 20 minutes
~ serve hot with slices of cheese on toast or garlic flavoured croutons

BAKED ONIONS

ingredients

4 large onions
1 oz., 25 g. or 2 tbsp. butter
2 oz., 50 g. or 1/2 cup grated cheese
1 tbsp. fresh chopped parsley
seasoning
a little cooked, chopped bacon (optional)

method

~ preheat oven to 350F, 180C or gas mark 4
~ peel the onions and trim the root end
~ place in an ovenproof dish with a little water and bake for about 1-1/2 hours until tender
~ scoop out the centre of each onion and chop finely
~ mix with grated cheese, butter, parsley and bacon, if using
~ season with a little pepper and spoon the stuffing back into the onion cases

~ return to the oven for about 15 minutes
~ serve hot

Tomato and Onion Salad

ingredients

4 firm tomatoes, finely sliced
3 medium onions, or 4 shallots, finely sliced
preferred dressing
a few chopped, mixed herbs

method

~ arrange tomato and onion slices on a serving dish and add preferred dressing
~ sprinkle with chopped, mixed herbs
~ chill for 10 minutes before serving

Cheese and Onion on Toast

ingredients

1 medium onion, sliced into rings
8 oz., 225 g. or 2 cups grated cheese
seasoning
a little milk
4 slices bread

method

~ boil onion rings in water for about 10 minutes and drain well
~ mix the cheese with seasoning and a little milk to make a thick paste
~ lightly toast one side of the bread under the grill
~ lay onion rings on the untoasted side and spread the cheese paste over the top
~ grill until golden brown
~ serve hot

Onions can be added to virtually any meal. Chop finely to add a little zing to the salad bowl, add to bolognaise or lasagne sauces, or finely slice and add to gravy to spice up a Sunday roast.

Parsley

Parsley can be used to garnish just about any dish you could imagine. Rather than throwing a sprig on a dish, chop finely and sprinkle over the food. It's much easier to eat like that.

Parsley Rice

ingredients

1 or 2 stalks celery, finely sliced
1 or 2 cloves of garlic, crushed
handful of chopped, fresh parsley
cooked rice
a little cooking oil

method

~ heat oil in a large pan and gently saute celery and garlic for 5 minutes, stirring constantly
~ stir rice and parsley into the pan and cook gently until heated

PARSLEY VEG

ingredients

handful of chopped parsley
a little butter
chosen vegetables (carrots, potatoes, etc.)

method

~ steam vegetables
~ drain well and return to the pan
~ add butter and parsley and mix well
~ serve hot

PARSLEY SOUP

ingredients

4 oz., 100 g. or 4 cups parsley, chopped
2 stalks celery, finely sliced
1 onion, chopped
1 tbsp. flour
1 oz., 25 g. or 2 tbsp. butter
1-1/2 pts., 900 ml. or 3-3/4 cups vegetable or chicken stock
seasoning

method

~ on a low heat, melt butter and cook celery and onion gently until starting to
   soften
~ stir in the flour and gradually add stock, stirring constantly
~ add parsley and seasoning and bring to the boil
~ reduce heat and simmer for about 20 minutes
~ allow to cool and blend in a liquidiser (blender) or food processor until
   smooth
~ reheat for a minute or two and serve hot
Drizzle a little cream into each bowl for an added touch of style

PARSLEY IDEAS

• Scrub and slice parsley root and add to stews and casseroles.
• Make a parsley sauce (see 'Chicory in Parsley Sauce' for details) as an
  accompaniment for many meals.
• Add to any salad bowl or salad dressing.
• Parsley pie, a traditional Cornish recipe, can be useful for using up leftovers. Almost
  fill a lightly greased pie dish with chopped parsley. Mix in any leftover, cooked lamb
  or other meat (cut into small pieces or minced). Add a couple of chopped
  hardboiled eggs, seasoning and pour stock over the whole lot. Cover with a pastry
  top and bake in a moderate oven 350F, 180C or gas mark 4 for about half an hour.

arsnip

Parsnips are a sweet-tasting, warm winter vegetable, and can be used in a variety of
recipes. Simply steam and toss in a little butter and mixed herbs or try one of these
recipes.

CURRIED PARSNIP SOUP

ingredients

2 lb., 900 g. or about 6 cups parsnips, peeled and finely chopped
2 oz., 50 g. or 4 tbsp. butter
1–2 onions, finely chopped
seasoning
2 to 2-1/2 pints, 1.1-1.5 litres or 5–6 cups vegetable or chicken stock
handful of fresh coriander (cilantro), chopped*
2 tsp. flour

* If coriander isn't available, use 2 tsp. curry powder, 1 tsp. cumin, and omit flour

method

~ melt butter in a large pan and gently cook onion and parsnip for a few minutes
~ stir in the curry powder and cumin or flour
~ slowly add stock
~ stir in the seasoning and coriander and bring to the boil
~ reduce heat and simmer for about 45–50 minutes until vegetables are tender
~ remove from the heat and allow to cool for a few minutes
~ blend in a liquidiser (blender) or food processor until smooth
~ return to the pan and reheat for a few minutes
~ serve hot

PARSNIP CRISPS

ingredients

young parsnips
vegetable oil
a little salt

method

~ peel parsnips and slice very thinly
~ deep fry in hot oil for about 3 minutes
~ drain on paper
~ re-fry for 1 minute and drain again
~ serve sprinkled with a little salt

PARSNIP BAKE

ingredients

2 lb., 1 kg. or about 6 cups parsnips
1 lb., 450 g. or 2-1/4 cups tomatoes
4 oz., 100 g. or 1 cup grated cheese
1/4 pint, 150 ml. or 1/2 cup vegetable or chicken stock
1/4 pint, 150 ml. or 1/2 cup single cream
3 tbsp. olive oil
1 tbsp. fresh coriander (cilantro), chopped
a little grated nutmeg
a little salt and black pepper

method

~ preheat oven to 325F, 170C or gas mark 3
~ peel parsnips and cut into thin slices
~ remove any hard core if using old parsnips
~ remove skin from tomatoes and slice (to loosen skin for easier peeling, put tomatoes into boiling water for about 30 seconds)

~ heat oil in a frying pan and fry parsnip slices for 2 minutes

~ place alternate layers of parsnip and tomato slices in a lightly greased casserole dish

~ sprinkle each layer with coriander, nutmeg, salt and pepper

~ mix cream with stock and pour over the vegetables

~ top with cheese and cover with lid or foil

~ bake for 45 minutes or until parsnip is tender

~ remove lid or foil for last 5 minutes of cooking time to brown top

~ serve hot

PARSNIP SALAD

ingredients

young parsnips

salad dressing, vinaigrette or other favoured dressing

seasoning

method

~ boil parsnips until just cooked, drain well and leave to cool

~ slice and place in serving dish

~ add salad dressing just before serving

Peas

Fresh-shelled peas can be eaten raw in salads and tossed into a stir-fry. Steam or boil until tender and serve them with any dish. Or add them to stews, casseroles or curries for extra bulk and nutritional value.

PEA SOUP

ingredients

2 lb., 900 g. or 8–9 cups peas, shelled

1 onion, finely chopped

2 oz., 50 g. or 4 tbsp. butter

1 handful of chopped, fresh mint

seasoning

2 pints, 1.1 litres or 5 cups chicken or vegetable stock

method

~ melt the butter in a large saucepan

~ add the onion and cook until soft

~ add the stock, peas, mint and seasoning

~ bring to the boil

~ reduce heat and simmer for 30–40 minutes

~ remove from heat and allow to cool slightly

~ blend in a liquidiser (blender) or food processor until smooth

~ return to pan and reheat for a minute or two

~ serve hot

PEAS AND CABBAGE

ingredients

half a firm cabbage, cut into fine slices

2 lb., 900 g. or 8–9 cups peas, shelled

10–12 spring onions or 3–4 shallots, sliced

1/4 pint, 150 ml. or 1/2 cup chicken or vegetable stock

method

2 oz., 50 g. or 4 tbsp. butter
seasoning
~ melt the butter in a large saucepan
~ add the rest of the ingredients
~ bring to the boil
~ reduce heat and simmer gently for around 20 minutes, until tender

Pea Guacamole

ingredients

12 oz., 350 g. or 3 cups shelled peas
1 or 2 cloves of garlic, crushed
2 spring onions, or 1 small shallot, chopped
handful of fresh coriander (cilantro), chopped
seasoning
1 tbsp. olive or nut oil
1 tsp. grated rind of a lime or lemon
juice of 1 lime or one half a lemon

method

~ steam or boil peas until tender and drain well
~ cool completely
~ put all ingredients into a liquidiser (blender) or food processor until smooth
~ chill before serving
~ serve with salad or on toast

Pea ideas

• Marrowfat peas can be boiled, mashed and served as 'mushy peas'.
• Mange tout or sugar snap peas are eaten with the pod. Serve in a salad or as a side dish tossed in an olive oil or walnut dressing.
• Peas can be added to stews, casseroles and curries. Try steaming them and tossing in a little butter and mint leaves.

Peppers

Bell peppers can be added to soups, stews, casseroles, ratatouille and bolognaise dishes. Chili peppers are perfect for spicing up any meal but should be handled with care. Always add sparingly.

Stuffed Peppers

ingredients

4 large red or green peppers
4 medium potatoes, peeled and diced
1 medium onion, finely chopped
3 tbsp. olive or nut oil
7 oz., 200 g. tuna, or cooked, chopped bacon
seasoning

method

~ cut the top off the peppers, scoop out the seeds and core
~ cook peppers and tops in boiling water for a few minutes
~ drain and allow to cool
~ steam diced potatoes until tender

~ allow to cool
~ mix together the tuna (or bacon), potatoes, onion, oil and seasoning
~ stuff each pepper with this mixture and replace tops on peppers
~ chill before serving or heat in a moderate oven (350F, 180C or gas mark 4) until hot

CHEESY PEPPER SLICES

ingredients

8 oz., 200 g. or 1 cup cottage cheese
4 oz., 100 g. or 1/2 cup cream cheese
1 tbsp. chopped chives
1 tbsp. chopped parsley
2 green or red peppers

method

~ cut off top of peppers, scoop out the seeds and core
~ mix together the rest of the ingredients until well blended and stuff the pepper cases
~ wrap in plastic film and refrigerate overnight
~ cut into thin slices and serve with a green salad

PEPPER SOUP

ingredients

1 green pepper, cored, be-seeded and chopped
1 red pepper, cored, be-seeded and chopped
a few slices of bacon
a little butter or cooking oil
3 or 4 tomatoes, chopped
1 onion, finely chopped
1 tbsp. flour
2 pints, 1.1 litres or 5 cups vegetable or chicken stock
seasoning

method

~ lightly grill bacon and cut into fairly small pieces
~ heat butter in a large pan and gently cook peppers, onion and tomatoes
~ stir in the flour and gradually add stock, stirring continuously
~ add the bacon
~ bring to the boil, then reduce heat and simmer for about 30 minutes until tender

RED PEPPER DRESSING

ingredients

1 red pepper, cored, de-seeded and chopped
olive or nut oil
1 clove garlic
1 tbsp. chopped parsley
a little wine or cider vinegar
seasoning

method

~ blanch pepper in boiling water for a few minutes, then remove skin and allow to cool
~ whisk the rest of the ingredients together and add the pepper
~ chill before serving

Pepper ideas

• Add peppers to any tomato dish, and throw a few mixed, chopped peppers in salads and stir-fry dishes.

Potatoes

Potatoes are probably one of the most versatile foods we can grow in our gardens. With a hungry family to feed, you can provide a different potato meal every day of the week. There are hundreds of potato recipes around, here are a few that will definitely encourage you into the kitchen.

Mediterranean Potatoes

ingredients

3 or 4 medium potatoes, scrubbed and diced (peel if desired)
1 courgette
1 green pepper
1 medium onion
a handful of fresh chopped herbs
juice of one lemon
a little olive or nut oil

method

~ steam potatoes until just cooked
~ drain and set aside
~ slice courgette, pepper and onion and gently saute in a little olive or nut oil until soft
~ stir in diced potatoes and herbs and cook gently for a few minutes
~ add lemon juice to the pan, stir and cook for a further minute
~ serve immediately

Cheesy Jackets

ingredients

medium baking potatoes
grated cheese
grated onion
mixed dried herbs
1 tbsp. olive oil

method

~ preheat oven to 375F, 190C or gas mark 5
~ pour olive oil in a baking dish and sprinkle on dried herbs
~ scrub and prick potatoes with a fork and bake in dish for around an hour
~ turn after half an hour to ensure a crisp, herby jacket to the potatoes
~ let sit for a few minutes after removing from oven
~ cut potatoes in half lengthwise and carefully scoop out the flesh into a mixing bowl
~ mash well and mix in cheese and onion
~ stuff the filling back into the potato skins and grill under a medium heat for 5–10 minutes
~ Bake more potatoes than you intend to eat, keep leftovers in the fridge overnight and slice and fry in olive oil the next day.

GARLIC POTATOES

ingredients

(add a little parsley to this potato recipe to keep the breath sweet)
3 or 4 large potatoes, well scrubbed
2–3 cloves garlic, crushed or finely chopped
butter
1/2 to 1 pint, 300–600 ml. or 1-1/4 to 2-1/2 cups of milk
2 oz., 50 g. or 1/2 cup grated cheese

method

~ preheat oven to 375F, 190C or gas mark 5
~ scrub and slice potatoes (peel if desired)
~ steam or boil until just cooked
~ with the butter, grease a deep, ovenproof dish
~ place slices of potato in layers into the dish, dotting with garlic
~ pour milk to half way up side of dish and sprinkle grated cheese on top
~ bake in centre of oven for around 25–30 minutes
~ serve hot

HOT POTATO LOAF

ingredients

2 lb., 900 g. or 5 cups potatoes, scrubbed and cubed (peel if desired)
4 oz., 100 g. or 1/2 cup cream cheese
3 large eggs
1/4 pint, 4 fl. oz. or 1/2 cup milk
1-1/2 tsp. salt
pepper
1 tsp. mixed herbs
1 tbsp. parmesan cheese

method

~ preheat oven to 375F, 190C or gas mark 5
~ cut potatoes into half-inch cubes (peel if desired)
~ parboil in boiling, salted water for 3 minutes
~ drain well
~ beat cream cheese until very soft
~ beat in eggs
~ stir in milk, salt, pepper, herbs and parmesan
~ spoon potato cubes into a prepared loaf pan and add cheese and egg mixture
~ cover with foil and bake for one hour
~ serve hot or cold

POTATO SALAD

ingredients

2 lb. or 1 kg. new potatoes (peel if desired)
4–6 spring onions, chopped finely
handful of chopped walnuts
3 fl. oz. or 75 ml. natural yoghurt
3 fl. oz. or 75 ml. mayonnaise
salt and black pepper

method

~ steam potatoes until just cooked, but not mushy
~ drain and cool completely
~ make a sauce by blending mayonnaise and natural yoghurt

~ when potatoes are cool, cut them into bite-sized pieces
~ mix in spring onions and walnuts and carefully stir in the sauce, coating all
  ingredients
~ chill for 30 minutes before serving

Pumpkin

Pumpkins are great to make Halloween lanterns, but the flesh can be enjoyed in
many different ways, in sweet and savoury dishes.

Roast Pumpkin

ingredients

I medium or half a large pumpkin
a handful of chopped mixed herbs
a little olive or nut oil

method

~ preheat oven to 375F, 190C or gas mark 5
~ pour a little oil into a baking pan
~ peel pumpkin and remove seeds
~ cut flesh into fairly large chunks and place in baking pan
~ pour a little oil over the top and sprinkle on the chopped herbs
~ bake in the oven for 30–45 minutes, turning once halfway through cooking
  time
~ pumpkin can also be roasted around a joint of meat (add to baking pan about
  45 minutes before end of cooking time)

Stir-fry Pumpkin

ingredients

I medium or half a large pumpkin
a handful of chopped coriander (cilantro)
a little olive or nut oil
I medium onion, chopped
I clove garlic, crushed
2 ripe tomatoes, chopped

method

~ peel pumpkin, remove seeds and cut flesh into small chunks
~ heat a little oil in a wok or large frying pan
~ cook onion and garlic for a few minutes, then add pumpkin, tomatoes and
  coriander
~ cook for a few minutes until all vegetables are tender
~ serve hot with rice

Spicy Pumpkin Soup

ingredients

2 lb., 900 g. or 6 cups pumpkin, peeled, seeds removed and sliced
2 or 3 leeks, trimmed and thinly sliced
2 oz., 50 g. or 4 tbsp. butter
a handful of chopped, fresh coriander (cilantro) and 2 tsp. flour OR 1–2 tsp.
  curry powder
2 pints, 1.1 litres or 5 cups vegetable or chicken stock

seasoning

a little natural yoghurt (optional)

method

~ heat butter in a large pan and cook leeks for a few minutes until starting to soften

~ add flour OR curry powder

~ stir well and cook for another minute

~ cut pumpkin into cubes and add to pan with stock, seasoning and coriander (if used)

~ bring to the boil, reduce heat and simmer for about 30–40 minutes until all vegetables are tender

~ allow to cool for a few minutes and blend in a liquidiser (blender) or food processor until smooth

~ return to pan, and reheat gently for a minute or two

~ swirl in a little natural yoghurt before serving to garnish, if desired

PUMPKIN TEA BREAD

ingredients

8 oz., 225 g. or 2 cups self-raising flour

4 oz., 100 g. or 1/2 cup butter

5 oz., 150 g. or 3/4 cup caster sugar

1 lb., 450 g. or 3 cups pumpkin flesh, sliced

2 eggs, beaten

6 oz., 175 g. or 1-1/2 cups chopped pecans or walnuts

3–4 tsp. cinnamon

method

~ preheat oven to 350F, 180C or gas mark 4

~ steam or boil pumpkin flesh until tender

~ press gently into a colander to drain as much water out as possible

~ allow to cool

~ beat all ingredients together except for the nuts (the mixture shouldn't be too soft – add a little more flour if necessary)

~ fold in the nuts

~ spoon mixture into a lightly greased 2 lb. or 1 kg. loaf pan and bake for about 1-1/2 hours

~ allow to cool on a wire rack

~ cut into slices

Raspberries

Raspberries are a delicate fruit with a unique and wonderful taste. They are packed full of vitamins and are one of the easiest fruits to grow in the home garden. Eat them straight from the plant for breakfast or try one of these wonderful recipes.

QUICK RASPBERRY PUDDING

ingredients

1 16 oz. or 425 g. can of rice pudding, or home-made rice pudding, cooled

8 oz., 225 g. or 2 cups fresh raspberries

method

~ keep a few raspberries for decoration and beat the remaining fruit with the rice pudding

~ pour into dessert bowls and decorate with the remaining raspberries

~ chill for a few minutes before serving

RASPBERRY MERINGUE

ingredients

3 egg whites

6 oz., 175 g. or 3/4 cup caster sugar

12 oz., 375 g. or 3 cups fresh raspberries

10 fl. oz., 300 ml. or 1-1/4 cups whipping cream

method

~ preheat oven to 225F, 110C or gas mark 1/4

~ cut an 8 inch (20.5 cm.) circle of greaseproof (wax) paper and place on a baking sheet

~ whisk the egg whites until stiff

~ gradually add half the sugar, whisking after each addition

~ fold in the rest of the sugar gently with a metal spoon

~ spread some of the meringue mixture over the circle of greaseproof paper, then make a fairly thick rim around the edge with the rest, to form a case

~ bake in the oven for about 2-1/2 to 3 hours until set but still white (if the meringue starts to go brown before it has set, leave the oven door slightly open for the rest of the cooking time)

~ remove from oven and allow to cool

~ put raspberries in the meringue case

~ whip the cream and pile on top of the raspberries

~ serve immediately

RASPBERRY JAM

ingredients

4 lbs., 1.8 kg. or 16 cups raspberries

4 lbs., 1.8 kg. or 8 cups sugar

this quantity makes about 6-1/2 lbs. or 3 kg. of jam

prepare jars in advance

method

~ prepare fruit: remove any leaf or stalks and damaged fruit

~ wash under gently running water and drain

~ place fruit in a large, heavy-based or preserving pan

~ bring to the boil, then lower the heat and simmer for about 20 minutes

~ stir from time to time to prevent sticking

~ make sure the fruit is very soft

~ remove from heat and stir in the sugar

~ keep stirring until sugar is dissolved

~ return to heat and boil rapidly for about 30 minutes

~ Test for a set: insert a sugar thermometer into jam. When the temperature is 221F or 105C the jam is ready. Remove any scum from the surface, leave to stand for 15 minutes then spoon the jam into prepared jars. Make sure the jars are warm before putting hot jam into them or the glass may crack.

RASPBERRY IDEAS

- Mash raspberries and use the puree to mix with ice cream or mix with a little water, cook gently and use the remaining sauce to pour over desserts.
- Use whole raspberries to decorate iced cakes or puddings.

Salsify

Not a very common vegetable these days, salsify is nutritious and warming. Add to stews and casseroles on chilly, winter days.

STEAMED SALSIFY

ingredients

salsify
a little butter
1 tbsp. mixed chopped herbs

method

~ peel or scrub salsify root
~ cut into required lengths
~ steam until tender
~ drain water and return to hot pan
~ add butter and herbs and gently stir until coated well
~ serve hot with any meal

SALSIFY FRITTERS

ingredients

1 lb. or 450 g. salsify
2 tbsp. thick cream
2 tbsp. natural Greek yoghurt
2 tbsp. corn flour (cornstarch)
seasoning
vegetable oil

method

~ peel or scrub salsify roots thoroughly
~ boil or steam for about 30 minutes or until tender
~ drain well and mash flesh roughly
~ mix in cream, yoghurt, corn flour (cornstarch) and seasoning
~ carefully drop teaspoons of the mixture into hot vegetable oil
~ fry until golden, turning once
~ drain on paper and serve immediately

SALSIFY WITH HOLLANDAISE SAUCE

ingredients

1 lb. or 450 g. salsify
3 tbsp. wine vinegar
6 black peppercorns
1 bay leaf
2 egg yolks
3 oz., 75 g. or 6 tbsp. butter
3 shallots, chopped
salt

method
~ wash and scrub salsify
~ cook in boiling water or steam until tender
~ drain, peel (if desired) and keep warm
~ put vinegar, shallots, bay leaf and peppercorns into a small saucepan
~ bring to the boil and simmer until volume is reduced by two thirds
~ cream egg yolks with half the butter and a pinch of salt in a small bowl
~ set over a pan of hot but not boiling water
~ strain vinegar mixture, add to egg yolks and whisk until thick
~ add rest of butter a little at a time, whisking after each addition
~ adjust seasoning
~ allow to cool slightly then pour over salsify and serve

SALSIFY IDEAS

• Use salsify to make a warming, winter soup. Or add to casseroles, one-pot recipes or even curries. To add to salads: steam or boil until just cooked, drain well, and allow to cool.

Spinach

Spinach is packed full of minerals and vitamins and can be cooked in a number of different ways. Young spinach leaves can be eaten uncooked in salads.

SPINACH AND BACON SALAD

ingredients
young spinach leaves
a few slices of bacon, grilled and chopped
1 small onion or shallot, finely chopped
croutons (optional)
Dressing
    3 tbsp. olive or walnut oil
    1 tbsp. wine or cider vinegar
    seasoning
    a little mustard

method
~ thinly slice spinach leaves and mix in a salad bowl with onions and cooled bacon
~ whisk all dressing ingredients together and pour over the salad
~ toss gently and add croutons if desired

EGGS FLORENTINE

ingredients
2 lb., 900 g. or 12 cups fresh spinach leaves
4 eggs
seasoning
Cheese sauce 1 oz., 25 g. or 1/4 cup flour
1 oz., 25 g. or 2 tbsp. butter
1/2 pt., 300 ml. or 1-1/4 cup milk
2 oz., 50 g. or 1/2 cup finely grated hard cheese
dash of powdered mustard
seasoning

method

~ steam or boil spinach until just cooked

~ drain, chop and place in an ovenproof dish

~ poach or lightly boil eggs and arrange on top of the spinach

~ melt butter in a pan and stir in the flour

~ stir over a low heat for a few minutes

~ remove the pan from the heat and very slowly stir in the milk

~ return to the heat and bring to the boil

~ reduce heat and simmer for 2 or 3 minutes until sauce thickens, stirring continuously to prevent lumps forming

~ remove from heat, season and quickly stir in grated cheese, stirring until cheese is melted

~ pour sauce over eggs and spinach

~ sprinkle a little extra cheese on top if preferred and grill under a moderate heat for a few minutes until brown on top

SPINACH SOUP

ingredients

1 lb., 450 g. or 6 cups fresh spinach, shredded

2 oz., 50 g. or 4 tbsp. butter

1 medium onion, finely chopped

1 oz., 25 g. or 1/4 cup flour

seasoning

1 pt., 450 ml. or 2-1/2 cups vegetable or chicken stock

method

~ melt the butter in a large saucepan

~ add the onion and cook until soft

~ stir in the flour

~ add the stock, spinach and seasoning

~ bring to the boil, reduce heat and simmer for 30–40 minutes

~ remove from heat and allow to cool slightly

~ blend in a liquidiser (blender) or food processor until smooth

~ return to pan and reheat for a minute or two

~ serve hot

SPINACH IDEAS

• Spinach pasta: if you make your own pasta, add finely chopped spinach to the dough to make 'pasta verde'. Or chop spinach leaves and add to any pasta dish. Add to a stir-fry or salad or steam lightly to serve as a side vegetable to accompany any meal.

Strawberries

Strawberries are another of the popular berries, used in flavourings, and many desserts. Try a few recipes with your own home-grown strawberries.

STRAWBERRY JAM

ingredients

3 lbs., 1.4 kg. or 6 cups strawberries, halved

3 lbs., 1.4 kg. or 6 cups sugar

juice of half a lemon

This quantity makes about 5 lbs. of jam (2.3 kg.). Prepare jars in advance.

method

~ prepare fruit: remove any leaf or stalks and damaged fruit

~ wash under gently running water and drain

~ place strawberries and lemon juice in a large, heavy-based or preserving pan

~ bring to the boil then lower the heat and simmer for about 20–30 minutes

~ stir from time to time to prevent sticking

~ make sure the fruit is very soft

~ remove from heat and stir in the sugar, stirring until sugar is dissolved

~ return to heat and boil rapidly for about 20 minutes

~ Test for a set: insert a sugar thermometer into jam. When the temperature is 221F or 105C the jam is ready. Remove any scum from the surface, leave to stand for 15 minutes then spoon the jam into prepared jars. Make sure the jars are warm before putting hot jam into them or the glass may crack.

STRAWBERRY AND ASPARAGUS

ingredients

12 oz., 350 g. or 3 cups asparagus

1 lb., 450 g. or 2 cups strawberries

2–4 oz., 50–100 g. or 1/2 to 1 cup pecan nuts, halved

1 small cucumber or half a large one

1/4 pint, 150 ml. or 1/2 cup mayonnaise or half mayonnaise and half natural yoghurt

method

~ cut asparagus into small lengths and steam or boil for about 5 minutes until just cooked

~ cool completely

~ prepare strawberries, removing all leaves and hulls

~ cut cucumber into slices or sticks

~ mix asparagus, strawberries, nuts and cucumber gently in a serving dish and refrigerate

~ serve cold with a mayonnaise sauce

STRAWBERRY IDEAS

• Make a juice for breakfast by blending strawberries and a ripe nectarine.

• Add strawberries to ice cream or other desserts.

• Chop a few strawberries and mix in with your morning cereal or muesli.

• Mix with other fruits to make an appetising fruit salad.

• Half fill a pie dish with strawberries. Sprinkle on a little sugar and top with a pastry topping or a crumble mix. Bake in the oven (350F, 180C or gas mark 4) for about half an hour.

• Sprinkle a little brown sugar on a bowl of strawberries and serve with whipped or double cream – lots of calories but great as an occasional treat.

Sunflower Seeds

Sunflower seeds are a delicious snack, and although gram for gram they are high in calories, there are many sunflower seeds to the kilo. Keep them in small sealed bags for long journeys. They are a healthy alternative to sweets and other processed snacks.

SUNFLOWER RICE

ingredients

3/4 pint, 40 ml. or 2 cups hot vegetable or chicken stock

8 oz., 200 g. or 1 cup basmati rice

3 oz., 70 g. or 1/2 cup of sunflower seeds

1 red pepper, de-seeded and sliced

1 onion, chopped

2 oz., 50 g. or 1/2 cup of peas

1 tsp. turmeric powder

1 tsp. cumin seeds

1/2 tsp. salt

1 tbsp. olive oil

handful of chopped fresh herbs (to garnish)

method

~ preheat oven to 400F, 200C or gas mark 6

~ heat oil and saute onion for 5 minutes

~ add cumin seeds and turmeric and saute for another minute

~ add rice and cook gently until translucent

~ add salt, red pepper and peas and cook for 2 minutes

~ add stock and sunflower seeds and bring to the boil

~ stir once and transfer to an ovenproof dish

~ cover and bake in oven for 20–25 minutes, or until rice has absorbed all liquid

~ sprinkle with chopped, fresh herbs before serving (optional)

SUNNY CHEESE BALLS

ingredients

4 oz., 100 g. or 1 cup grated cheese

4 oz., 100 g. or 1/2 cup cream cheese

4 oz., 100 g. or 2/3 cup of roasted sunflower seed kernels

1 small, finely chopped red or green pepper, deseeded

method

~ remove cheeses from refrigerator at least an hour before using and blend together

~ blanch chopped pepper in boiling water for a couple of minutes until soft

~ drain well, and leave to cool

~ when cool, stir pepper into cheese mixture and blend in a food processor or beat until pepper is mixed well

~ roll into about 24 balls and refrigerate for 30 minutes

~ remove from fridge and roll in sunflower seed kernels

~ chill for at least 2 hours

Cabbage and Seed Salad

ingredients

12 oz., 300 g. or 3 cups shredded cabbage

1–2 oz., 25–50 g. or 1/4 to 1/2 cup chopped onion

1 large tomato, chopped

3–4 slices cooked bacon, chopped

1–2 oz., 25–50 g. or 1/4 cup roasted sunflower seed kernels (no salt)

1–2 oz., 25–50 g. or 1/4 to 1/2 cup feta cheese, cut into small cubes

add preferred salad dressing

method

~ combine all ingredients in a large serving dish, and pour dressing on just before serving

Banana Seed Cakes

ingredients

2 small to medium bananas, very ripe

6 oz., 150 g. or 1-1/2 cups self-raising flour (if using plain flour, add 1–2 tsp. baking powder)

3 oz., 75 g. or 1/3 cup sugar

3 oz., 75 g. or 6 tbsp. butter

5–6 oz., 125–150 g. or 1 cup sunflower seed kernels

method

~ preheat oven to 350F, 180C or gas mark 4

~ peel and mash bananas

~ in a large bowl, cream butter and beat in sugar and bananas

~ mix flour with sunflower seeds and baking powder (if used)

~ fold the flour mixture into the banana mix and stir together well

~ put tablespoons of dough onto an ungreased baking sheet leaving about 2 in. (5 cm.) between them

~ bake for around 15 minutes, or until just starting to brown

Sweet Corn

The most popular way of eating corn on the cob is by boiling or steaming it until tender and serving with butter. Cobs can also be grilled, roasted or popped on the barbeque. To remove kernels from cob, hold cob upright on a chopping board and scrape kernels off with a sharp knife.

Corn Fritters

ingredients

12 oz. or 2 cups cooked corn kernels

1 medium finely chopped onion

4 oz., 100 g. or 1 cup flour

2 eggs

a little milk

seasoning

cooking oil

Batter:

method

~ put flour into a bowl, make a well in the centre and break both eggs into it
~ add a little milk and beat well until smooth
~ heat cooking oil in a pan and saute onion until soft, then remove from heat
~ stir corn kernels, onion and seasoning into batter mix
~ fry spoonfuls of mixture in hot oil until golden brown
~ drain on paper and serve hot or cold

CORN VEGGIE BURGERS

ingredients

cooked corn kernels
breadcrumbs
chopped herbs
1 egg
flour
cooking oil

method

~ mix cooked corn kernels with a few breadcrumbs and chopped herbs
~ stir in a raw, beaten egg to bind the mixture together
~ shape into burgers
~ dredge with a little flour and grill or fry

This is a basic recipe but any of the following ingredients could be added:

~ finely chopped onion, sweet peppers or chili peppers
~ fresh, chopped coriander (cilantro)
~ tsp. of curry or chili powder
~ cut chives
~ cooked peas
~ diced, cooked potato
~ mashed potato can be used to replace breadcrumbs
~ chopped, fresh or canned tomato
~ sliced mushrooms

Search around for any leftovers and create your own family recipe.

CORN PILAF

ingredients

4 cups cooked rice
2 oz., 50 g. or 4 tbsp. butter
12 oz., 300 g. or 2 cups sweet corn kernels
1 onion, finely chopped
4–6 slices of bacon, chopped
4 oz., 100 g. or 1-1/2 cups mushrooms, sliced
2 oz., 50 g. or 1/2 cup grated cheese
2–3 sliced tomatoes
seasoning

method

~ cook the rice while you prepare other ingredients and keep hot
~ melt the butter in a wok or large frying pan
~ saute the onion until soft
~ add the bacon and mushrooms and cook until bacon is crisp
~ add the corn and seasoning and heat for a further minute or two

~ add the cooked rice

~ cook for a few minutes stirring gently to avoid burning

~ stir in the cheese at the last minute and put mixture into a warmed, serving dish

~ garnish with sliced tomatoes and serve immediately

BAKED SWEET CORN

ingredients

4 corn cobs, prepared for cooking

3 oz., 75 g. or 6 tbsp. melted butter or olive oil if preferred

1–2 tbsp. fresh chopped thyme

seasoning

method

~ preheat oven to 325F, 160C or gas mark 3

~ steam or boil the corn in water for a few minutes and drain well

~ place each cob on a sheet of foil

~ mix thyme and seasoning into melted butter or oil and pour gently over each cob

~ wrap loosely in the foil, but make sure each 'packet is sealed to keep the flavours in

~ bake for 10–15 minutes in the oven or until corn is tender

~ serve immediately

Tomatoes

Next to onions, tomatoes must be the most widely used food in the kitchen and they keep all their goodness when cooked. Experiment, especially if you have a good crop in the garden. There's nothing like the taste of a home grown tomato!

SUMMER TOMATO SOUP

ingredients

2 lb., 900 g. or about 5 cups tomatoes (when chopped)

1 onion, finely chopped

1 medium potato, diced

2 oz., 50 g. or 4 tbsp. butter

seasoning

1–2 tsp. finely chopped fresh basil

1–2 pts., 900 ml. or 2-1/2 to 5 cups vegetable or chicken stock

method

~ melt the butter in a large pan

~ saute the diced potato and chopped onion until soft

~ keep on a low heat and stir to avoid burning

~ peel tomatoes by plunging them into boiling water for a few seconds to loosen the skin

~ cut into quarters

~ add tomatoes, stock and seasoning to the pan, stir and bring to the boil

~ reduce heat and simmer for about 30 minutes

~ add basil and cook for a further 5 minutes

~ serve immediately, or sieve or blend until smooth and reheat for a minute or two

STUFFED TOMATOES

ingredients

4 large tomatoes
a little cooking oil
1 onion, finely chopped
4 slices of cooked bacon, chopped
a handful of mixed herbs
4 oz., 100 g. or 1-1/2 cups sliced mushrooms
1–2 oz., 25–50 g. or 1/3 cup ground nuts
2–4 oz., 50–100 g. or 1/2 to 1 cup grated cheese
seasoning

method

~ preheat oven to 350F, 180C or gas mark 4
~ slice the top off each tomato and scoop out the seeds
~ place tomatoes in a greased, ovenproof dish
~ heat the cooking oil in a frying pan
~ cook the onion and mushrooms for a few minutes
~ add the rest of the ingredients and stir together until well mixed
~ remove from heat and spoon the mixture into the four tomato shells
~ put the tops back on the tomatoes and bake in the oven for about 20 minutes, until hot
~ serve immediately

PARMESAN BAKED TOMATOES

ingredients

fairly firm tomatoes
grated parmesan cheese
a handful of fresh, chopped basil
a little cooking oil

method

~ preheat oven to 350F, 180C or gas mark 4
~ pour a little cooking oil into an ovenproof dish and heat for a minute or two
~ cut tomatoes in half and place cut side up in the baking dish
~ sprinkle chopped basil over the tomatoes
~ top each one with a spoonful of grated parmesan
~ bake for about 20 minutes or until tomatoes are hot and cheese has melted
~ serve hot

TOMATO IDEAS

• Use fresh tomatoes where you would normally use tinned. Use as a base for bolognaise and chilli sauces.
• Chop tomatoes in chunks, add to cooked pasta with grated cheese on top and bake in the oven for 10 minutes or so.
• Add finely chopped tomatoes to the salad bowl.
• Slice and add to a stir-fry.
• Fresh basil is perfect with tomatoes. Slice a few firm tomatoes, sprinkle with chopped basil and chill for a few minutes before serving.

Turnip Greens

Turnip greens can be used instead of spinach in most recipes, although they are sometimes slightly bitter and are tastier when cooked.

Butter and Garlic Greens

ingredients

turnip greens
1–2 cloves garlic, crushed
a little butter

method

~ steam greens until tender
~ drain well then chop finely
~ return to pan and stir in butter and crushed garlic cloves
~ serve hot

Spring Veg Stir-fry

ingredients

2 tbsp. olive or nut oil
1–2 cloves garlic, finely chopped
1 onion, or 3–4 spring onions, chopped
6 oz., 150 g. or 1-1/2 cups asparagus, cut into small lengths
8 oz. or 200 g. young carrots
6–8 oz., 150–200 g. or 2 cups turnip greens, shredded
12 oz., 350 g. or 2 cups broccoli florets
4 oz. or 100 g. mange tout (snow peas)
juice of half a lemon, or if preferred 1–2 tbsp. apple juice
a handful of chopped, fresh, mixed herbs

method

~ heat oil in a wok or large frying pan
~ fry garlic and onion for a few minutes
~ add the rest of the vegetables and stir over a medium heat until just tender
~ add a little water to the pan if needed
~ add juice and herbs and cook for a further minute or two
~ serve hot
Use any spring vegetables you have available for this dish.

Braised Turnip Greens with Chestnuts

ingredients

1-1/2 lb., 700 g. or 6 cups turnip greens, chopped
1 lb., 450 g. or 3-1/2 cups peeled chestnuts
1 oz., 25 g. or 2 tbsp. butter
6 shallots, sliced
2 sticks celery, sliced
1/2 pint, 300 ml. or 1-1/4 cups chicken or vegetable stock
4 oz., 100 g. or 1/2 cup cooked, chopped bacon (to garnish)
1 tbsp. chopped fresh parsley (to garnish)

method

~ preheat oven to 325F, 170C or gas mark 3
~ put chestnuts in a saucepan and cover with half the stock
~ add a small piece of the butter and simmer until chestnuts are soft

~ melt remaining butter in a pan and gently cook shallots and celery for 2 minutes

~ put turnip greens, chestnuts, shallots and celery in a casserole dish and pour the remaining stock over

~ cover and bake for about 40 minutes, or until vegetables are tender

~ serve garnished with bacon and parsley

SPICED TURNIP GREENS AND POTATOES

ingredients

I lb., 450 g. or 2-1/2 cups potatoes, chopped and peeled (if desired)

I lb., 450 g. or 4 cups turnip greens, finely chopped

I large onion, chopped

a little chopped, fresh ginger

2 cloves of garlic, finely chopped

I chopped fresh green chilli

I tsp. coriander powder, or I tbsp. fresh chopped coriander (cilantro)

2 crushed cardamom pods

1/2 tsp. garam masala

salt to taste

a little lemon juice

2 tbsp. sunflower oil

method

~ heat oil in a large pan and gently saute onion, garlic and ginger for a few minutes

~ add chilli and spices and cook for another 2 minutes

~ add potatoes and saute until nearly cooked

~ add greens and cook with the lid on until potatoes are finished cooking

~ add a little water if too dry or starting to stick to the pan

~ taste and season with a little salt and lemon juice if desired

~ serve hot

Watercress

Watercress is strong in taste as well as nutrients and doesn't have to be grown in running water. Make the most of your home-grown watercress and try these tasty recipes.

WATERCRESS AND PASTA SOUP

ingredients

I oz., 25 g. or 2 tbsp. butter

2 onions, chopped

2 bunches of watercress, finely chopped

2-1/2 pints, 1.3 litres or 5–6 cups chicken or vegetable stock

seasoning

3 oz., 75 g. or I cup spaghetti or vermicelli, broken into short lengths

method

~ heat butter in a large pan and cook onion until soft

~ add stock, watercress and seasoning

~ bring to the boil, reduce heat and simmer for about 20 minutes

~ stir in the pasta and simmer a further 5–10 minutes until it is tender

~ serve hot

GREEN SALAD

ingredients

1 bunch of watercress
lettuce leaves
1 green pepper
4–6 spring onions
half a lemon

method

~ wash and chop watercress, discarding any tough stalks

~ wash lettuce and shred finely

~ chop spring onions into small pieces

~ remove core and seeds from green pepper and slice into rings

~ put watercress, lettuce, onions and pepper into serving dish and mix gently together

~ slice lemon finely and arrange on top of salad

~ serve chilled with a dressing

BASIC VINAIGRETTE DRESSING

ingredients

1 tbsp. wine or cider vinegar
1 tsp. mustard
a little salt and black pepper
2 tbsp. nut or olive oil

method

~ whisk all ingredients together

~ taste and adjust seasonings as desired

WATERCRESS IDEAS

• Make a herb bread – use Garlic Bread recipe, but use chopped watercress instead of garlic and parsley.

• Add chopped watercress to stews and casseroles.

• Use sprigs of watercress to garnish any dish.

Edible Flowers

Edible flowers are a stylish addition to any meal. The Romans used them to garnish their banquets 2000 years ago. There are hundreds of edible flowers, wild and cultivated. Here are a few to look out for in your garden. Use them to garnish your wonderful garden recipes.

Broccoli ~ after the broccoli floret comes the flowers. Leave a few on the plant and use the tiny yellow flowers in a stir-fry and salad

Carnations ~ add to wine, sweets, and use as cake decorations

Dandelions ~ use flowers to make a tasty and healthy jam

Elderflower ~ make elderflower champagne from the flowers. Make it non-alcoholic for a refreshing summer drink (and good for you)

Honeysuckle ~ flowers taste of honey and can be eaten raw and added to wines and desserts. Honeysuckle berries are highly poisonous – DO NOT EAT

Jasmine ~ jasmine flowers are normally used to make tea. Simply steep the flowers in boiling water and strain.

Nasturtium ~ colourful flowers add a peppery tang to the salad bowl as well as making it look nice

Roses ~ Rose petals can be used to garnish desserts, flavour ice cream or add to jams. Rose hips (a great source of vitamin C) can be made into rose hip syrup or wine.

Violets ~ Sprinkle a few violet flowers into a salad. They have a slightly perfumed taste. Violet flowers are traditionally crystallised and used as cake decorations.

Resources

All tables compiled from the Nutrient Data Base USA: http://www.nal.usda.gov

Other useful places to find nutritional data:

Australian Sites:

Active Healthy Lifestyles – www.helpguide.org/life/healthy_eating_diet.htm
Department of Health – www.health.wa.gov.au/health_topics/n/nutrition.cfm
Dieticians Association of Australia – www.daa.asn.au
Food Down Under – www.fooddownunder.com
Food Standards – www.foodstandards.gov.au
Food Watch – www.foodwatch.com.au
Health & Medical Research Council – www.nhmrc.gov.au/publications/index.htm
Healthy Active Australia – www.healthyactive.gov.au
Healthy Eating Club – www.healthyeatingclub.org
Nutrition Australia – www.nutritionaustralia.org
Vegetarian/Vegan Society of Queensland – www.vegsoc.org.au
Well Being – www.wellbeing.com.au

UK and European Sites:

5 A Day – www.5aday.nhs.uk
BBC Healthy Living – www.bbc.co.uk/health/healthy_living
British Dietetic Association – www.bda.uk.com
British Nutrition Foundation – www.nutrition.org.uk
Eat Well – www.eatwell.gov.uk
European Food Information Council – www.eufic.org
Food Standards Agency – www.food.gov.uk
Mind, Body and Soul – www.mindbodysoul.gov.uk
Net Doctor – www.netdoctor.co.uk
Nutrition Society – www.nutritionsociety.org
Vegetarian Society of the UK – www.vegsoc.org
Wired For Health – www.wiredforhealth.gov.uk

American and Canadian Sites:

American Autoimmune Related Diseases Association – www.aarda.org
American Dietetic Association – www.eatright.org
Council for Responsible Nutrition – www.crnusa.org
Health Castle – www.healthcastle.com
Linus Pauling Institute – http://lpi.oregonstate.edu/infocenter

National Women's Health Network – www.womenshealthnetwork.org
Nutrition Data – www.nutritiondata.com
Office of Dietary Supplements – http://ods.od.nih.gov/index.aspx
Pyramid Plan – www.mypyramid.gov
US Food and Drug Administration – www.fda.gov
World's Healthiest Foods – www.whfoods.com
West Virginia Dietetic Association – www.wvda.org

Plant Information:

BBC Gardening – www.bbc.co.uk/gardening
Botanical – www.botanical.com
Divine Energy Spirit – www.divineenergyspirit.com/Herbs.htm
Drying Foods – www.ag.uiuc.edu/vista/html_pubs/DRYING/dryfood.html
Flower and Garden – www.flower-and-garden-tips.com
Garden Action – www.gardenaction.co.uk
Garden Guides – www.gardenguides.com
Mushroom Council (US) – www.mushroomcouncil.org
National Gardening Association – www.garden.org
The Foody – http://thefoody.com
Think Vegetables – www.thinkvegetables.co.uk

Index